Radiation Protection in the X-ray Department

To my dear husband Peter and wonderful daughters Erica and Lianna, who have all had to share me with this book for the last 18 months.

Radiation Protection in the X-ray Department

Simone Plaut HDCR(R) FETC

Radiation Protection Co-ordinator,
Central Middlesex Hospital Trust,
London

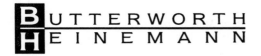

Butterworth-Heinemann Ltd
Linacre House, Jordan Hill, Oxford OX2 8DP

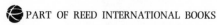 PART OF REED INTERNATIONAL BOOKS

OXFORD   LONDON   BOSTON
MUNICH   NEW DELHI   SINGAPORE   SYDNEY
TOKYO   TORONTO   WELLINGTON

First published 1993

British Library Cataloguing in Publication Data
Plaut, Simone R.
  Radiation Protection in the X-ray
  Department
  I. Title
  616.07

ISBN 0 7506 0606 1

Library of Congress Cataloguing in Publication Data
Plaut, Simone.
  Radiation protection in the x-ray department/Simone Plaut.
  p. cm.
  Includes bibliographical references and index.
  ISBN 0 7506 0606 1
  1. Radiography, Medical – Safety measures – Handbooks, manuals,
  etc.
  I. Title.
  [DNLM: 1. Radiation Dosage. 2. Radiation Injuries – prevention
  and control. 3. Radiation Protection – methods. WN 650 P721r]
  RC78.3.P53   92–49239
  616.07′57′0289–dc20   CIP

Typeset by Lasertext Ltd., Stretford, Manchester
Printed and bound in Great Britain by Biddles Ltd
Guildford and King's Lynn

Contents

Foreword

Global warming, the depletion of the ozone layer, car exhaust emissions, use of fossil fuels and large-scale farm use of pesticides: all are 'health' issues of which the general public has now become aware. The issue which strikes the greatest fear is however that of radiation and in particular the radiation associated with nuclear power plants and X-rays. This fear is understandable even if it is not logical: the 'nuclear discussion' has been 'going public' for nearly fifty years whereas most other pollutants have reached the public arena only during the last decade. It is also true that radiation hazards are the most well-documented and have probably had the greatest exposure in the scientific and lay press. The medical profession has long been a user of ionizing radiation and can certainly lay claim to being the largest contributor to man-made radiation burdens in the individual. With this dubious claim to fame and the enhanced public awareness of the effects of radiation on health, it is important that all in the profession take steps to minimize the radiation doses received and to ensure that the public understands the risks associated with medical X-rays. This handbook is intended to help the radiological profession do just that: reduce doses and educate the public.

The most important individual in this dose-reduction and educational exercise is the radiographer. It is he or she who is in closest contact with the patient during the study and, in the majority of examinations, is the one to 'press the button'. Radiographers are therefore charged with the task of acting in the most professional way possible, using the latest scientific results and techniques in order to reduce doses and explaining to the lay person what hazard the radiation presents and the measures that have been taken to reduce it during the examination. To do this effectively they must be well-informed. This handbook contains information they need and in a form they can use. The author is eminently suited to write this handbook. As an experienced radiographer she has all the practical details to give; as an experienced radiation adviser she is fully conversant with radiation protection practice and the latest research results. The text covers some of the basics of radiation dosimetry, the terminology that is used, and summarizes safe radiation practice and the doses received. It is a book that should occupy a place in every radiographer's pocket and on the bookshelves of all diagnostic radiation users.

Robert Speller
University College London

Preface

This book is intended to fill a gap in the range of books available on radiation protection within diagnostic radiology. There is no single reference book to answer the increasingly frequent and exacting questions from the public on the safety of their X-ray examination, less still a small handbook that can be carried around in the radiographer's pocket.

Most of the currently available books on the subject are written by physicists and consequently approach the material from a scientific rather than a purely practical viewpoint. Much use is made of mathematics and mathematical notation, which can be off-putting to the unfamiliar reader.

There are many excellent books available to the general public on the subject of radiation risks and hazards, but these tend to be evaluating those from the nuclear power industry or the Chernobyl disaster, and the discussions of radioactivity are confusing to anyone attempting to grasp the salient points of diagnostic X-ray protection, where by comparison, far lower radiation doses are involved.

The reference books available giving radiation dose data can be difficult to comprehend when dipping into them for the first time. They necessarily contain much scientific data, which may not be useful to a radiographer or radiologist searching for a specific dose figure for submission to a patient or junior hospital doctor.

This book attempts to provide the information most often requested by radiographers and radiologists about radiation protection, in an easily accessible form. It explains the terms commonly used in the subject. There are easy-to-comprehend tables of organ doses from common X-ray examinations and comparative risks from everyday activities such as smoking or driving a car. In addition there is information on the risks to a fetus from diagnostic X-ray procedures.

This book is written for radiographers and radiologists

(especially those studying for the Fellowship of the Royal College of Radiologists Part One exam) using a wide range of current research data and containing all the information necessary to satisfy the core of knowledge requirements. It will also provide a practical guide to junior physicists on the type and level of information required by hospital professionals.

Acknowledgements

I am not an expert in all these areas, and have had to rely on the generous help of a number of people, especially:

- Mr Barry Wall of the National Radiological Protection Board for reading the manuscript and making a number of useful suggestions. Both Barry Wall and Paul Shrimpton, also of the NRPB, have always known the answers to my tricky questions, and have sent me copies of their excellent publications.
- Dr Anna Thornton of St Mary's Hospital, London, for her enormous input and support.
- Dr Alan Calverd for his excellent help on several of the chapters.

Without the input of these and others, this book would not have been published.

I would also like to thank the following people who have encouraged me in my career and writing: 'Prem' Premachandra, Phil Shorvon, Carol Cornish and all my colleagues at Central Middlesex Hospital, Adrienne Finch of Hatfield University, Robert Speller for encouragement and guidance, David Thomson for being a tremendously supportive RPA, and, again, Alan Calverd who has been inspirational.

1

Exposure, dose, LET, kerma: the jargon jungle

People are often bewildered by an array of radiation dosimetric quantities and units. To complicate matters further, new units have been introduced in line with the SI system. A useful quantity, the röntgen, a measure of exposure, is no longer used for legal purposes. The old units are still to be found in most American and Soviet publications, in older textbooks and on pieces of radiation-measuring equipment (many of which are manufactured in the USA).

This chapter will attempt to explain these quantities and units, what each is used for, which old units they replace, and provide some analogies from everyday life to help in understanding them. *Note:* length is a quantity, feet are units.

Exposure

Exposure is a measure of the ionization produced in air by X radiation. Units are coulombs per kilogram (C/kg); formerly the röntgen(2.58×10^{-4} C/kg).

Absorbed dose

Absorbed dose is measured in gray (Gy), and is the base unit of radiation dose. This unit is named after the British physicist Hal Gray who died in 1956. He studied under Rutherford in Cambridge, then undertook pioneering work in dosimetry, particularly in the evaluation of absorbed dose from ionization chamber data. He was the originator of the Bragg–Gray relationship, the basis of most radiotherapy dosimetry. He later worked at Mount Vernon Hospital, near London, on radiotherapy cancer research.

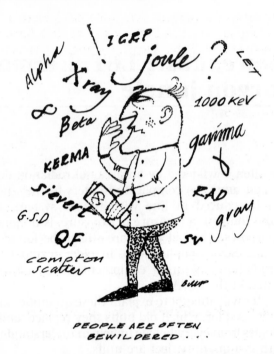

PEOPLE ARE OFTEN
BEWILDERED . . .

The radiation energy absorbed by the patient is measured in grays. *One gray deposits one joule of energy in a kilogram of irradiated tissue.*

Absorbed dose makes no distinction between different types of radiation (some of which are more hazardous than others) or between types of tissue or organ irradiated (some of which are more sensitive to radiation damage than others). Absorbed dose is commonly reported in terms of centigrays in radiotherapy departments. The predecessor of the gray, the rad is exactly equal to one-hundredth of a gray – hence the term centigray. Had it not been possible to make such an easy transition between the rad and the gray, accidental over- or underirradiations might have occurred in radiotherapy departments during the changeover period.

1 rad = 0.01 Gy
1 rem = 0.01 sievert (Sv)

An absorbed dose in grays does not give a full picture of the possible harm to the patient. One joule per kilogram of energy absorbed from sunshine, a bath or the central heating makes you feel good. One joule per kilogram of ionizing radiation (1 Gy) will make you sterile.

Dose equivalent

Dose equivalent is measured in sieverts, after the Swedish physicist, Rolf Sievert. This unit allows the damage capability of a quantity of radiation to be expressed in a single number, thus giving a guide to the risk. The former unit was the rem.

The biological effects of alpha particles and neutrons are far greater than that from diagnostic-range X radiation. For this reason a correction or quality factor (QF) is used to convert absorbed dose (in grays) to dose equivalent (in sieverts). It is the photon dose that would have the same biological effect.

Quality factors for different types of radiation

The 1990 recommendations of the International Commission on Radiological Protection (ICRP).
Beta particles, X-rays and gamma-rays QF = 1
Neutrons < 10 keV QF = 5
Neutrons 10–100 keV QF = 10
Neutrons 100 keV–2 MeV QF = 20
Neutrons > 20 MeV QF = 5
Alpha particles QF = 20

- 1 Gy of beta particles, X-rays or gamma-rays gives a dose equivalent to 1 Sv.
- 1 Gy of low-energy neutrons gives a dose equivalent of 5.0 Sv.
- 1 Gy of 50 keV neutrons gives a dose equivalent of 10.0 Sv.
- 1 Gy of alpha particles gives a dose equivalent of 20.0 Sv.

Absorbed dose (in gray) and dose equivalent (in sieverts) are numerically equivalent for diagnostic-range X radiation.
The conversion of sieverts to rems is 1 Sv = 100 rem.

The sievert is a large unit and thus in diagnostic dosimetry, the dose equivalents are usually given in mSv, or thousandths of a sievert.

Alpha particles are more highly ionizing than X-rays and so for the same number of grays your 'goose would be cooked' more quickly (see also LET later in this chapter).

The different quality factors reflect the various biological effects in tissue. Alpha particles and neutrons are heavy and strongly ionizing. When passing through a medium, they cause intense ionization over a short path, losing all their kinetic energy to cause ionization events. All the damage (broken chemical bonds) occurs within a tiny volume, reducing the capacity for repair. This characteristic of ionizing radiation is called linear energy transfer (LET).

Linear energy transfer

Radiation is often described in terms of low or high LET. LET is a measure of how the energy of a photon or particle is distributed along its path. LET is defined as the total energy deposited in an absorber per unit path length. LET can also be expressed as the number of ion pairs per unit length of path.

As the ionizing radiation or particle moves through a medium, such as tissue, atoms become ionized. The amount of energy needed per ionization event depends upon the binding energy of the electron concerned, but is reasonably constant in tissue. Because of their great mass, alpha particles move slowly through tissue, and the double positive charge is extremely attractive to electrons. Neutrons are also heavy, and travel slowly. Neutrons are electrically neutral and so do not cause direct ionization. None the less, they produce intense ionization by causing the ejection of protons from atomic nuclei, and by causing other nuclei to recoil. The LET for both alpha particles and neutrons is high, since a large number of ions will be produced per unit distance travelled.

Beta particles, X-rays and gamma-rays have low or zero mass. They move quickly through tissue, and cause fewer ionization events per unit path length.

A 1 MeV alpha particle can travel 5×10^{-6} m in tissue, before coming to a stop due to lack of energy.

An electron can travel up to 5×10^{-3} m in tissue, finally stopping for lack of energy.

Alpha particles produce $\simeq 1000$ ion pairs per μm travelled in tissue.

X-, gamma- and beta-rays produce $\simeq 100$ ion pairs per μm travelled in tissue.

Effect of ionization on the cell

The concentration of ionization events in a small volume of tissue will affect the ability of cells to self-repair. If many molecules are affected in one cell, that cell is less likely to continue its normal function. It may die, lose functional ability, lose its reproductive function or it may become cancerous. If many cells are affected in one organ, that whole organ or body system may fail. It is this mechanism which causes radiation-induced bone marrow failure in radiation victims.

This subject is covered in greater detail in Chapter 2.

Weighting factors for different tissues of the body

One Gy of absorbed dose does *not* have the same risk wherever it is delivered in the body. The various tissues have weighting factors, as described below. These have also been reviewed in the 1990 ICRP recommendations and both the old and new figures are quoted in Table 1.1.

The 1990 ICRP recommendations allow for the numbers of non-fatal as well as fatal cancers induced due to radiation exposure. The anguish and misery caused to sufferers from non-fatal cancers and the corresponding costs in terms of health care expenditure are reflected in these weighting factors. These recommendations indicate what emphasis should be placed on radiation protection, and allow a comparison of money to be spent on caring for radiation-induced cancer patients versus the cost of techniques for radiation dose reduction and equipment.

The risk of malignancy per sievert is not the same for the various tissues of the body. It is lower for the thyroid than for the lung, but the highest single organ weighting factor is for the gonads, where hereditary damage as well as malignancy must be allowed for.

These weighting factors are calculated by reference to experi-

Table 1.1 WEIGHTING FACTORS FOR DIFFERENT BODY TISSUES, ACCORDING TO ICRP 1977 AND 1990 RECOMMENDATIONS

Tissue or organ	Weighting factors	
	ICRP (26) 1977	ICRP (60) 1990
Testes and ovaries	0.25	0.20
Breast	0.15	0.05
Bladder		0.05
Red bone marrow	0.12	0.12
Colon		0.12
Lung	0.12	0.12
Stomach		0.12
Thyroid	0.03	0.05
Liver		0.05
Oesophagus		0.05
Bone surfaces	0.03	0.02
Remainder	0.30	0.05

Remainder refers to all organs or tissues not listed separately.

mental as well as the Hiroshima and Nagasaki survivors data. The later factors (ICRP, 1990) are the most appropriate, as they incorporate the recent re-evaluation of these data, and are believed to be more realistic.

Effective dose equivalent

Application of these weighting factors and summing them for the organs irradiated gives the quantity: *effective dose equivalent* (renamed effective dose when using 1990 weighting factors). This quantity takes into account the differing radiosensitivities of the body tissues. To draw a cooking analogy, it allows the difference between stewing steak and raw egg to be considered; the amount of energy required for a perfect scrambled egg will leave the stewing steak inedible.

The effective dose equivalent also allows a range of non-uniform organ and tissue doses to be combined as a single number. Broadly speaking, this number represents the risk to health for the irradiated person, regardless of the widely different dose equivalents received by the organs of the body.

It also allows comparisons to be made between the risk to health from different types of examination, such as computed tomography (CT) scanning and plain radiography of the same body part, where the organ doses are quite different.

A 5 mSv effective dose equivalent has the same potential health detriment regardless of how the patient received it, be it from a number of chest X-rays, a CT scan or a technetium study. The use of effective dose equivalent only relates to moderate doses, and possible late effects. Potentially lethal doses and chronic radiation-induced disease as studied in radiobiology cannot be described in this way.

Collective effective dose equivalent

It is sometimes of value to have a measure of the total dose of radiation to an entire population. Here it is instructive to compare doses from natural background radiation to those received from occupational exposure. This is done by multiplying average effective dose by the number of people in the population.

For example, the average annual natural effective dose in the UK is 1.9 mSv (or 1.9×10^{-3} Sv). If the UK total population is approximately 57 million, then the collective effective dose to the whole community is:

$$1.9 \times 10^{-3} \times 57 \times 10^6 = 1.1 \times 10^5 \, \text{man Sv}$$

With occupational exposure, very much smaller numbers of people are exposed. For example, the average doses received by medical workers in the UK are $\simeq 0.7$ mSv per year. This multiplied by the 39 000 such workers in the country gives a total collective effective dose for this group of:

$$0.7 \times 10^{-3} \times 39\,000 = 27.3 \, \text{man Sv}$$

The impact of radiation doses received by medical workers is clearly negligible in comparison with background radiation doses received by the entire population, which includes children.

The hierarchy of dose quantities

Absorbed dose (energy imparted by the radiation to unit mass of tissue)
↓
Dose equivalent (absorbed dose weighted for harm from different radiations)
↓
Effective dose (dose equivalent weighted for radiation sensitivity of different tissues)
↓
Collective effective dose (dose equivalent to a population)

Example of an effective dose calculation

Suppose a patient received effective doses to the following:
100 mSv to the lung
70 mSv to the liver
300 mSv to the bone surfaces
The effective dose is calculated using the tissue weighting factors quoted above, giving:

$$(100 \times 0.12) + (70 \times 0.05) + (300 \times 0.02) =$$
$$12 + 3.5 + 6 \, mSv = 21.5 \, mSv$$

This is the same overall risk to the patient's health regardless of whether he or she received that dose uniformly throughout the whole body.

Genetically significant dose (GSD)

This is the radiation dose received by the gonads of the patient, but with a weighting factor depending on the expected future number of children that that person might produce – the possible effect dependent on the remaining fertility of the individual.

Postmenopausal women do not receive any GSD but for men there is no upper limit.

Table 1.2 EFFECTIVE ATOMIC NUMBERS OF DIFFER-
ENT BODY TISSUES

Material	Effective atomic number (Z effective)
Bone	11.6
Muscle	7.4
Fat	6.3
Water	7.4
Air	7.6

Attenuation processes – photoelectric absorption and Compton scatter

Photoelectric absorption occurs when an incoming photon of ionizing radiation is absorbed by an electron of an atom in the absorber. If the incoming photon has sufficient energy, the electron may be ejected from its atom and travel off as a photoelectron. This electron is a charged particle and will cause further ionization within the absorber until it has used up its kinetic energy. The kinetic energy will be what remained from the original photon of ionizing radiation less the energy used in releasing the electron from an atom.

This process predominates at lower energies because X-ray photons are more efficient at ejecting electrons when the binding energy of the electron is close to that of the incoming photon of radiation. The extent of photoelectric absorption is proportional to the cube of the atomic number of the material. This explains the radiographic contrast seen between bone and soft tissue, since the average atomic number of bone is greater than that of soft tissue.

Photoelectric absorption is proportional to (atomic number)^3. The effective atomic number of a material is the average of the atomic numbers of the constituent atoms weighted for their relative amounts. Examples are given in Table 1.2. From these values, it is clear that most of the differences are small, particularly between water and air. In radiography of the lung, fluid may be difficult to see when compared with air. Water close to muscle (such as a cyst) may be indistinguishable. Water is an excellent muscle-equivalent phantom material (Fig. 1.1). The dose distribution with p.e. absorption is superficial, giving higher skin doses.

Compton scatter occurs when the energy of the incoming

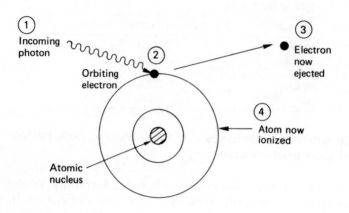

Fig. 1.1 Photoelectric absorption.

ionizing radiation photon is much greater than the binding energy of electrons in the absorber. All the electrons now behave as if unbound and undergo billiard-ball type collisions with incoming photons. The original photon goes off at an angle, and with reduced energy. The recoil electron also goes off at an angle with the remainder of the photon energy. The electron may travel only in the forward direction; the photon may travel in any direction, including backwards. The extent of Compton scatter is proportional to electron density in an absorber, hence dense materials cause more. Barium sulphate and lead are both extremely dense materials – bone less so, hence the loss of radiographic contrast at higher kilovoltages. Tissues of similar atomic number but different density, e.g. water and air, are better visualized at higher kilovoltage settings. This is the rationale behind high-kilovoltage chest radiography (Fig. 1.2). Compton scattered radiation distributes the dose deeper in the body than photoelectric absorption, sparing the skin, but even affecting organs outside the original irradiated area.

Note: Kerma is not as useful or important a quantity as those defined above. It has been included for completeness, but the busy reader is advised to go to Chapter 2.

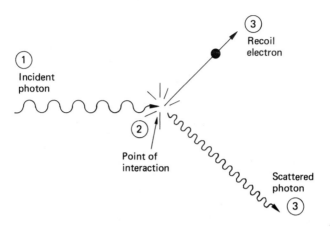

Fig. 1.2 Compton scatter.

Kerma

Kerma is a measure of the absorption of radiation in a small mass a medium, i.e. the number of photoelectric and Compton events. It is no different to absorbed dose (which measures total energy absorbed in the medium) except for higher energy radiations, not encountered in diagnostic radiology. Higher energy radiations produce energetic electrons which could in turn cause ionization remote from the irradiated area, and thus cannot be part of the original small mass under consideration. Kerma approximately replaces the quantity 'exposure'. It is best thought of as 'the dose to the air' and is usually measured with an air-filled ionization chamber.

The name *kerma* is derived from *k*inetic *e*nergy *r*eleased per unit *m*ass of tissue by indirectly ionizing radiation; that is, anything that is not a charged particle. Use of this quantity implies that no secondary radiation is produced within the patient; the energy is transferred to electrons already present in the tissue. Kerma can be quantified with X-rays, gamma-rays and uncharged neutrons, but not with charged particles (alpha,

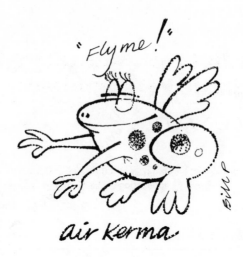

air kerma

beta or protons). In the diagnostic X-ray energy range, air kerma is equal to absorbed dose in air. The gray replaces the röntgen.

Air kerma of 1 Gy is equal to an absorbed dose in air of 1 Gy.

1 R = air kerma of 8.7 mGy.

1 Gy = 115 R.

2
How radiation interacts with tissue: basic radiobiology

The first section of this chapter is revision; the familiar reader may wish to go directly to 'ionization in the cell nucleus', below.

Action of ionizing radiation

Ionizing radiation can cause damage when it passes through tissue because it deposits its energy in that tissue. The energy of the photon of radiation causes ionization; that is, electrons are removed from atoms. Atoms are linked to each other to form molecules, bonded by the outer shell electrons. Remove such an electron, and that bond is broken (Fig. 2.1).

Consider this ionization event has occurred within a cell.

The effect of an ionization event such as that above will depend upon where in the cell it occurred.

Function of DNA (Fig. 2.2)

Deoxyribonucleic acid or DNA is the cell database, the medium in which all information is stored. It acts as a blueprint for the preparation of proteins by the cell. These proteins in turn control the function of the cell both as an individual unit and as part of the whole body.

The atoms of the DNA molecule are arranged in a paired spiral staircase structure. (The DNA is not normally seen in individual chromosomes except during cell division. Chromosomes are composed of coiled coils of DNA molecules.) Linking the two staircases are pairs of organic bases whose names are cytosine, guanine, thymine and adenine (C, G, T and A).

A sequence of just three of these bases codes for a specific

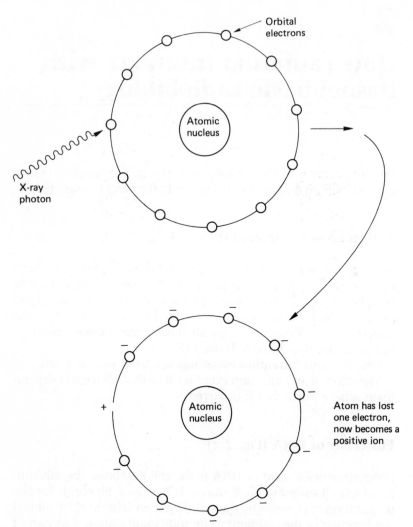

Fig. 2.1 Atom undergoing ionization.

amino acid. (There are 20 such amino acids found in human cells. Proteins are composed of long chains of amino acids arranged in a specific sequence.) The order in which the coding bases appears tells the cell how to compose proteins, with full stops to tell it where to finish.

The cell nucleus contains all the genetic material.

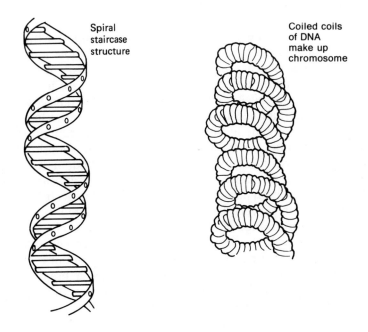

Spiral staircase structure

Coiled coils of DNA make up chromosome

Fig. 2.2 The structure of DNA.

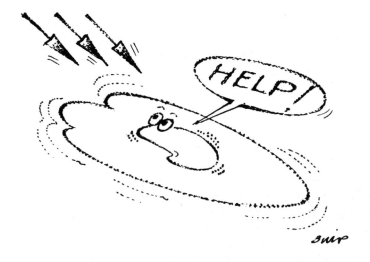

Ionization in the cell nucleus

Proteins include the enzymes and hormones upon which the whole function of any cell and ultimately the whole individual depends. The accuracy of information on the DNA in the cells is vital to the continued health of the individual. An inability to make even one specific enzyme can be a fatal illness for the sufferer. DNA damage to reproductive cells can interfere with the accuracy of genetic function, resulting in disruption to the future generation. Such damage is called a *mutation*. Mutations can be recessive or dominant, or can occur at random. Recessive mutations are far more common but usually appear in the offspring only if both parents pass on the mutant gene. Inbreeding of a population or very large numbers of irradiated individuals makes the appearance of affected children more likely.

Alternatively high doses can kill reproductive cells causing temporary or even permanent sterility. The arrival of a photon of ionizing radiation can be enough to cause a break in the staircase of DNA. If this breakage is on both sides of the molecule then it cannot self-repair. In such a case a piece of DNA may be lost from the chromosome.

It may alternatively rejoin incorrectly with unpredictable results. Such damage repeated several times can result in a *chromosome aberration*.

The more radiation received by the cell, the more likely such damage is to occur. People who have received even modest doses of radiation continuously have been found to have chromosome aberrations in the blood. Some chemotherapy agents are also capable of causing such changes to chromosomes.

Genes and cancer

Another mechanism by which neoplastic (cancerous) change is believed to take place is the activation of oncogenes. These are mutant genes present in some individuals. They can be activated or 'switched on' by the action of ionizing radiation or certain chemical agents. Some are inserted by a virus.

Once activated, the mutant gene causes cell replication to occur unchecked, forming a tumour or leukaemia. Other genes are also known to play a part in cancerous change: suppressor genes stop oncogenes from being expressed; repair genes can repair damage, loss of these results in radiosensitivity; checkpoint genes halt cells in G2 stage and check for damage before mitosis.

Ionization within the cytoplasm

A large proportion of the cell is composed of water (up to 80%). This is therefore where most of the interactions will occur. The arrival of ionizing radiation may cause a water molecule to lose an electron forming:

$$H_2O \rightarrow H_2O^+ + e^-$$

The positive ion dissociates into a hydrogen ion and an uncharged species called a free radical or OH. If two OH radicals join together they can form hydrogen peroxide – H_2O_2. This is a powerful and toxic oxidant (or bleach) which can damage the cell and its DNA if produced in large enough quantities. Hydrogen peroxide is produced deliberately in the liver where it is used to break up proteins, but here speedy neutralization by enzymes can avoid its toxic effects.

Ionization effects on cell membranes

The membrane of a cell is important to many aspects of function. The function of the kidney, for example, depends almost entirely on the ability of cells to retain differing permeabilities to certain electrolytes. It is believed that ionizing radiation may damage the cells' ability to act as a barrier to particular ions, thus interfering with cell function. For example, nerve cells maintain a potential difference across their membranes by the use of different levels of sodium and potassium inside and outside the cell. If this ability is lost the cell ceases to perform its function properly.

Action of very large doses

The cell can be affected adversely in many ways by the arrival of photons of ionizing radiation. Very large doses are not seen in diagnostic radiology, but it is still useful to be aware of the effects of such doses.

A large radiation dose may kill a cell. A lower dose may sterilize the cell so that it continues to function but can no longer reproduce itself when necessary. Lower doses may temporarily suppress the cell's ability to reproduce, with recovery at a later stage. There may be induction of cancer, seen perhaps only many years later. Some cells within the body have a very high turnover rate and need to be continually replaced to maintain organ function. For example, the intestinal mucosal lining requires constant replacement. If a very large dose of radiation is received, these cells may become sterile and unable to reproduce. With the death of existing cells and no replacements, the intestinal lining will rupture and slough away. Bacteria can then cross the gut wall, causing septicaemia and even death.

In the brain, the action of very large doses of radiation will cause massive oedema (swelling) of the brain tissues, due to failure of the membranes to maintain their ionic balance, and rupture of small blood vessels.

The red blood corpuscles have no nucleus and cannot reproduce. They are produced in the red bone marrow and live for about 6 weeks. A very heavy radiation dose may knock out the active (red) bone marrow. Once all the victim's existing red cells are dead, massive blood transfusions and a bone marrow transplant will be needed for survival.

People who have received potentially lethal doses of radiation survive for differing periods depending upon the total dose absorbed, and the overall percentage of organs and systems receiving sufficient radiation to destroy their function. The final variable is different people's inherent genetic susceptibility to radiation. Many Hiroshima and Nagasaki bomb victims received similar large doses, with widely differing results: some died, some developed cancer, and some survived unaffected.

Such levels of dose *cannot* be received in normal circumstances during radiotherapy, let alone diagnostic X-ray procedures. Even in a case where a unit failed to terminate a radiographic exposure, the X-ray tube would probably overheat and fail before a dangerous dose could be delivered. Nevertheless it is vital that radiographers are vigilant and watch control panel mA meters for any sign that an exposure has failed to terminate. For both patient care and image quality, the disappearance of the mA

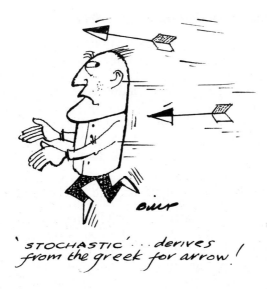

'STOCHASTIC'... derives
from the greek for arrow!

meter from most diagnostic X-ray unit designs is a detrimental step.

Stochastic and non-stochastic effects

Stochastic effects

These are the only type of effect likely to be seen in diagnostic radiology. They are chance effects. The word stochastic derives from the Greek for arrow. 'It gets you or it doesn't'. These effects are due to cell damage rather than cell death and there may be a long period between the irradiation and the manifestation of the effect – in some cases as long as 20 or 30 years. This delay is called the latent period. There is no clear threshold and different individuals have different likelihoods of sustaining injury.

The overall risk for a large group is dependent on size of dose received.

Possible effects included are induction of solid cancers and leukaemias, and genetic alteration to future generations. Not all these effects are detrimental; the genetic mutations caused by cosmic radiations over the millennia have enabled evolution of the species to take place.

Non-stochastic or deterministic effects

Non-chance effects are more likely than stochastic effects to be due to cell death or irreparable damage than to genetic mutation. They are the basis of radiotherapy and are seen only in the individual who received the radiation dose (or exceptionally, in a fetus present *in utero* at the time of the irradiation). Non-stochastic effects include cataract formation (2–5 Sv or more), sterility (temporary: 0.1 Sv lasts for approximately 1 year; 2.5 Sv lasts 3 years or more, or is possibly permanent) and hair loss (3 Sv or more).

Deterministic effects are less easily quantifiable, and include growth and mental retardation in children.

These effects can be extremely useful: some leukaemia patients undergo a treatment known as total body irradiation. A potentially lethal dose of irradiation (7–10 Gy $\simeq$ 2–5 Sv) is used to kill off deliberately their (diseased) red bone marrow, followed by a bone marrow transplant and intensive reverse-barrier nursing to prevent infection while donor marrow 'takes' and the patient recovers.

How high is high? (Note: these are whole-body doses)

20 Sv: death occurs within hours due to central nervous system damage.

5–10 Sv: death occurs within days due to gastrointestinal radiation sickness. (Stem cells in the gut are killed; the gut lining cannot be replaced, as it is constantly sloughed away; haemorrhage occurs. Bacteria are able to enter the blood from the gut, causing septicaemia.)

2–5 Sv: death occurs within weeks due to bone marrow failure.

The amount of radiation that would kill 50% of individuals within 60 days, or $LD_{50/60}$ for radiation in healthy adults receiving good medical care is 3–5 Sv.

Annual occupational exposure of 5×10^{-3} S(mSv) corresponds to an annual risk of cancer induction of 8×10^{-5} (8 in 100 000 people).

How does this compare with the doses given in diagnostic radiology (Table 2.1)? (The effective doses given in various examinations are given in more detail in Chapter 4.)

Table 2.1 EFFECTIVE DOSES GIVEN IN DIAG-
NOSTIC RADIOLOGY

Area of treatment	Effective dose ($\times\ 10^{-3}\,$Sv)
X-ray	
Posteroanterior chest	0.02
Anteroposterior abdomen	1.0
Barium meal	3.8
Barium enema	7.7
CT	
Chest	9.0
Abdomen and pelvis	9.5
Lumbar spine	6.0

Note: these doses are to part of the body only.

How can we compare the doses given in diagnostic radiology with the very high doses known to cause death or serious injury? There is a multitude of data on large doses, from various sources such as Hiroshima and Nagasaki atomic bomb survivors, radium dial painters (who licked their brushes and ingested radium) and uranium miners (who inhaled large quantities of radon gas in the mines). Fewer data are available on small doses because the numbers of affected subjects for a given level of irradiation will be small. It thus becomes difficult to pick out radiation-induced effects over and above naturally occurring disease rates. Vast populations are required to assess effects and this makes research prohibitively expensive.

Much of the low-dose data is based on extensive research using small laboratory animals, where short reproductive cycles make them highly suitable for such studies. Radiation effects in various mammalian embryos have greater similarities than the effects of most other teratogens or embryopathic agents. This is because radiation has a direct effect on the developing embryo, and variations in placental transport or maternal metabolism do not significantly alter the results of radiation experiments with pregnant mammals, unlike those experiments using any other teratogen (Brent, 1989). Rabbits are three times more radiation-resistant than humans: in a large-scale nuclear war, rabbits could survive in great numbers.

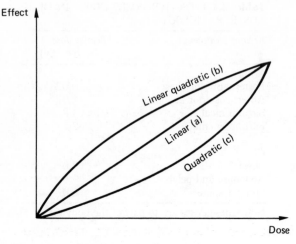

Fig. 2.3 Dose-effect models.

Dose–effect models

Various models (graphs) of calculated deductions have been drawn up to predict the effects at the lower levels of dose, as seen in diagnostic radiology. There are three main models (Fig. 2.3);

1. Linear – a straight-line graph, no threshold: double dose = double risk.
2. Linear quadratic – a basic straight line with a partial curve; small effects are seen at lower doses. Much greater numbers are affected as the dose rises. High L.E.T. radiation.
3. Quadratic – a pronounced curve, flat initially, becoming steeper. Effects are extremely small until a threshold is reached, when there is a marked increase in the numbers affected.

Which is the correct model? No one is certain. It is even possible that different people or ethnic groups follow different curves (see Chapter 3 for more information).

3
Ionizing radiation risks and how to assess them

The damaging effects of ionizing radiation

This chapter compares the risks from some everyday activities with those from radiation. There then follows a short discussion of the enormous differences between perceived and actual risk.

Much of our knowledge of the harmful effects of ionizing radiation is from the follow-up of atomic bomb survivors of the attacks on Hiroshima and Nagasaki during World War II. The doses received varied from microsieverts to tens of sieverts and the effects on the population have been subject to continuous review and intensive research. There has also been much data from patients who received radiotherapy for non-malignant conditions such as ankylosing spondylitis and scalp ringworm. Before the availability of ultrasound, many babies were X-rayed *in utero* for various complications of pregnancy, such as twin gestation and breech presentation, neither of which is known to carry an increased risk of cancer. Graphs have been drawn and estimates made of how the very high doses, for which we have ample data, can be translated into a risk for the much smaller doses received in modern diagnostic radiology, for which data are sparse.

In Chapter 2 we saw how ionizing radiation can cause tissue damage, how it can interfere with the cell cycle, cause premature ageing and even neoplastic (or cancerous) changes. In order to appreciate the risks to health due to exposure to radiation we must first understand something about risks, how they are described and how we perceive them.

Risk and hazard

When a major plane crash occurs some potential travellers become frightened and may even cancel their holidays. Aeroplanes however remain an extremely safe way to travel; it is simply our perception of risk that has changed. For all of us, the death rate is 100%. Death is not a preventable occurrence. However, by careful adjustment of our lifestyle, we can tip the balance in favour of death due to old age rather than some other earlier method.

Tobacco and alcohol are addictive and carcinogenic and would not receive approval today as foodstuffs or medicine, yet we continue to use both in vast quantities, despite the certain knowledge that they damage our health.

Hazard: A set of circumstances which may cause harmful consequences.

Risk: The likelihood of the harmful consequences caused by the hazard.

How do we assess risk? Counting deaths is one way, but non-fatal disease or serious injury can severely damage quality of life and must be included. Even an injury from which the sufferer fully recovers leaves consequences in terms of lowered promotion prospects and detriment to social or family life.

When seatbelt laws were introduced there appeared to be an increase in the severity of crash injuries. Cynics claimed that the seatbelts caused an increase in the number of injuries. In fact, the explanation for the shift was rather more complex.

1. Some moderate injuries prevented altogether by the seatbelt were not seen at all in casualty.
2. Some people who would have died if they had not been wearing seatbelts survived severe road accidents and so did not go direct to the mortuary.
3. There was no change in side impacts.

Congenitally deformed babies, sterile adults and non-fatal cancers all cause great personal problems for sufferers and their families, yet do not appear in the mortality statistics. To quote only the number of deaths caused is misleading and does not truly reflect the other consequences of radiation exposure.

Relative contributory factors to deaths in the UK

Smoking 10 cigarettes a day	1 in 200
All natural causes – aged 40	1 in 850
Flu (all ages)	1 in 5000
Accident on the road	1 in 8000
Radiation dose of 10 mSv effective dose equivalent	1 in 10 000
Leukaemia	1 in 12 500
Accident at work	1 in 43 500
Radiation (for workers in the nuclear industry)	1 in 57 000
Being hit by lightning	1 in 10 000 000
Release of radioactivity from a nuclear power station	1 in 10 000 000

For activities over which we have no choice, we all expect the risks to be exceedingly low. With the use of medicines, patients will accept a degree of risk, because some benefit is gained.

For voluntary actions, such as drinking, smoking, drug abuse and dangerous driving – these all carry risks, yet we seem content to make these choices.

Main causes of death

The main cause of death in the UK is cardiovascular disease. If we reduce obesity and fat intake, atherosclerosis risks are markedly reduced. Smoking 15 cigarettes a day doubles the risk of coronary heart disease. The relative risk for young people is much higher; the most susceptible individuals die at an early age.

Cancer

This disease carries an unreasonable fear, and for many years was a taboo subject. Cancer is not a new disease; there are cases described in the Old Testament. Despite many scare stories in the press, the rates of cancer are steady, with only skin cancer on the increase (probably due to overexposure to the sun and ozone layer depletion. In Victorian times when a pale skin was fashionable, skin cancer rates were far lower than today).

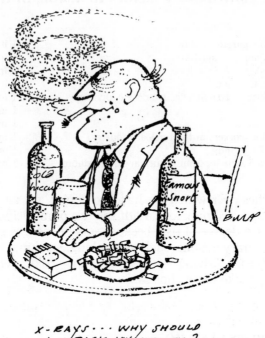

X-RAYS... WHY SHOULD
I RISK MY HEALTH?

Cancer rates appear to rise when other causes of death are reduced. Many postmortems on elderly people reveal asymptomatic cancers, unrelated to the cause of death. Cancer appears to be part of the ageing process.

The death rate from lung cancer amongst women is on the increase, and this appears to be due to the increase in smoking amongst women. Some women feel that smoking helps in weight control. There must be safer ways to diet!

The small numbers of additional cancers caused by particular products or pollutants may be difficult to quantify when there are already large numbers of naturally occurring cancers. A researcher setting out to prove a link can be apparently successful if he or she chooses the population carefully, since clusters of sufferers from a particular disease occur naturally in any case, especially if a family group who are naturally susceptible is included. This type of study, sensationalized in the media, causes an unwarranted fear of the disease and yet a quick perusal of

Table 3.1 RISKS OF CANCER DUE TO VARIOUS FACTORS

Variable	Risk of cancer
Tobacco	30%
Poor diet	35%
(Some foods are known to be carcinogenic. Low-fibre diets increase the risk of colonic cancer)	
Alcohol	3%
Pollution	2%
Food additives	< 1%
Sexual practice	7%
(Cervical cancer; multiple partners: the risks can be reduced by circumcision/use of condoms)	
Occupation	4%
Medicines	1%
Geophysical (e.g. sun)	3%
Infection (e.g. HIV)	10% and rising (AIDS)

Table 3.1 reveals the self-destructive way in which many of us fall prey to cancers.

Radiation causes terror, yet in small doses can be similar in carcinogenicity to smoked foods; however, people do not run in terror from pastrami or kippers!

Radiation can cause damage, but careful consideration must be given for a full understanding. Prior to 1950, radiologists

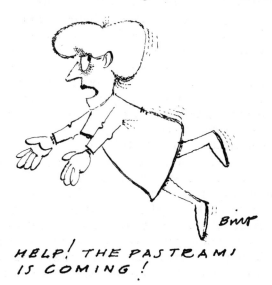

HELP! THE PASTRAMI IS COMING!

Table 3.2 TYPICAL RISKS FROM X-RAY EXAMINATIONS (PER 10^6)

Examination	Hereditary effect		Effect on fetus	
	Paternal irradiation	*Maternal irradiation*	*Childhood cancer*	*Mental retardation*
Lumbar spine	0.2	16	200	1560
Abdomen	2.0	11	170	1300
Pelvis	24	6.3	100	740
Intravenous urogram	23	19	220	1610
Barium meal	0.8	9.4	220	1620
Barium enema	5.4	26	960	7200

were allowed to receive 1 mSv per day; then it was noticed that many radiologists who had been in the profession since the early 1920s had an elevated cancer rate compared to other doctors. Safety measures were introduced, and the cancer rates amongst radiologists are now no higher than for other medical personnel. The increase in interventional radiology has raised the exposure rates amongst radiologists, and early cataracts have been seen in some individuals. Eye protection is vital for such work. Lead glasses are available for as little as the cost of a good pair of sunglasses.

Of the Hiroshima and Nagasaki survivors, only 1% died from radiation-induced leukaemias in the 30 years post exposure. Another 3% died from other radiation-induced cancers. A pattern seems to emerge – some individuals are more susceptible to radiation-induced cancers than others. Safety limits are fixed at a level that will protect the most susceptible, even though this may be well below any risk increase for the majority of the population. Table 3.2 shows the typical risks of hereditary and fetal effects from various X-ray procedures.

If 1 million people receive 10 mSv effective dose equivalent, 100 extra deaths (over the normal incidence) will occur. To put this into perspective, however, in the UK there is currently a 22% chance (averaged over all ages) of death from cancer. If you receive a 10 mSv effective dose equivalent of ionizing radiation to your whole body, the risk goes up to 22.01%. Are we not unreasonably fearful? A quick reference to Chapter 4 will reveal which examinations impart effective dose equivalents of 10 mSv or more (in brief, these are intravenous urograms, barium meal and enema, and computed tomography scans.

Interventional radiology carries even higher doses, but is performed to treat life-threatening conditions, justifying the increased risk). For workers in the nuclear industry, the average dose is 1.4 mSv per year, giving an average risk of cancer *lower* than the risk of fatal accidents in all other industries.

Mutations

Many of the women who were pregnant in Hiroshima and Nagasaki during the dropping of the atom bombs lost their babies. Some of those who were in early pregnancy went on to give birth to deformed babies. These abnormalities are classified as congenital (postconception), not genetic (inherited).

There is no discernible elevated risk for babies conceived after the atom bomb attacks on Japan in all the 45 years since World War II. Perhaps it is still too early to see those mutations expressed in the descendents of the survivors, or perhaps the risks are lower than we fear. (See Chapter 7 for more information on risks to pregnant women.)

Background radiation

The average dose equivalent for members of the UK population is 2.5 mSv per year, of which 0.1–1.0 mSv is due to building materials. The rest is from cosmic radiation and other external sources.

Doses are at the higher end of the range in Cornwall and parts of Scotland due to granite in the ground and building materials. In poorly ventilated granite buildings the levels can exceed 50 mSv per year, as a result of radon gas build-up. Advice is available from the National Radiological Protection Board on this in the UK (and the local equivalent elsewhere); the Board can provide dosimeters to measure radon gas levels in homes and offices where there is concern.

Radon has a short half-life (3.5 days) and improved ventilation or use of a sump under the floorboards can reduce risks considerably. The sump absorbs the radon, a pump blows the air out and dumps it away from the house.

In much of the rest of the world background levels are lower than those seen in the UK. The usual average is 0.7 mSv. Some places however do have considerably higher levels. Examples are the Monazite sands in Kerala state, southern India. Here background doses may be as high as 4–5 mSv per year. The inhabitants have been studied extensively and do show slightly increased levels of chromosome aberrations compared to control groups.

In Iowa and Illinois in the USA the levels of radioactivity in the drinking water are higher than elsewhere, giving a high background radiation dose. The levels of bone cancer seen in the inhabitants is elevated, but is lower than in Chicago which has no radioactivity in the drinking water.

Cosmic radiation is one of the constituents of background radiation and is due to extraterrestrial phenomena.

Supersonic aircraft, such as Concorde, fly at higher altitudes than other aeroplanes, and carry a radiation meter on board. If the radiation dose rates rise above a predetermined level, the craft will drop to a lower altitude, and must reduce to subsonic speeds.

The Chernobyl nuclear power station accident in April 1986 caused enormous concern. Hysteria, whipped up by the media using headlines such as 'The worst accident in the world' (Hawkes et al., 1986), caused us to imagine an occurrence of world-shattering proportions. Many unfortunate Ukrainians have been killed or severely injured by this tragic accident, but for most of Europe the background radiation rose by between 3 and 5% for that year, with smaller rises for subsequent years.

Total background radiation may be responsible for 1000 of the 140 000 naturally occurring deaths due to cancer each year in the UK. Chernobyl may have caused 100 or so more. This is far fewer than deaths due to smoking, road accidents and alcohol abuse.

- Less than 1% of cancer deaths are due to background radiation.
- Less than 0.1% are due to medical uses.
- Less than 0.001% are due to non-medical artificial sources such as the nuclear power industry and weapons testing, yet the public are most frightened of this last tiny value.

Cancer risk could be reduced by encouraging people to follow these simple guidelines:

- Drink alcohol in moderation.
- Stop smoking (avoid passive smoking?).
- Improve your diet and adopt a healthier lifestyle.
- Sunbathe in moderation, and never without a sunscreen.
- Reduce the number of sexual partners – never have unprotected sex.
- Reduce the radon levels at home.
- *And then* start reducing medical radiation exposure.

Safer sex – then safer X-rays.

4

Radiation doses in radiology

Medical X-rays represent by far the largest manmade source of public exposure to ionizing radiation. There is considerable evidence that substantial reductions in these medical exposures are possible without detriment to patient care. The Ionising Radiation Regulations 1988 called for:

1. Patient doses to be in accordance with accepted diagnostic practice.
2. Patient doses to be as low as reasonably practicable to achieve the required purpose.
3. Professionals directing medical exposures to be familiar with typical doses, their means of measurement and reduction.

Typical radiation doses given to patients during routine X-ray examinations are given in the tables in this chapter. The values are mainly those from NRPB R200, published by the National Radiological Protection Board (NRPB) and based on a national UK survey of 20 randomly selected hospitals published in 1986. The figures given are mean values recorded by the survey and reflect what could be considered as a benchmark for good practice. All our hospitals should aim to use mean or average doses which at least match, or preferably undercut, the radiation doses quoted in these tables.

In many examinations, the range of doses delivered for the same procedure varied greatly between centres – by a factor of 10 or more in several instances, e.g. minimum of 0.83 mGy; mean of 9.19 mGy; maximum of 59.10 mGy (entrance skin dose for the lumbar spine examination: NRPB R200). Whilst some of this variation is due to patient size, much is due to poor technique, poor equipment, poor maintenance, failure to employ gonad and breast protection or use of outdated technology (non-use of rare earth screens etc.). Some of the remedy lies in the hands of the radiographer and his or her manager. Radiography performed properly is a very low-risk procedure; done improperly it may not be so.

To verify the level of doses delivered to patients, simple methods are readily available. These include use of thermoluminescent dosimeters attached to the patient's skin surface, and use of dose–area product meters. Careful selection of patient size is required to exclude this variable from affecting results. For further information, the interested reader is referred to the *National Protocol for Patient Dose Measurements in Diagnostic Radiology*; report of the dosimetry working party of the Institute of Physical Sciences in Medicine and published by them in December 1992.

In order to simplify Table 4.1, some of the organ doses, the standard deviations, maximum and minimum doses which formed part of the original report have been omitted. The interested reader should consult NRPB R200.

Examinations not included in NRPB R200

The technique, number of films and screening times vary enormously between centres and even between individual radiologists at the same centre. Rough estimates can be derived by adding the dose from the fluoroscopic screening time (Table 4.2) and doses for the radiographic exposures, and reaching a total.
Micturating cystogram: see protocol in your department.
Small bowel enema: see protocol in your department.
Note: exact details of these examinations vary enormously between centres.

Readily available, inexpensive personal monitoring dosimeters can be used to ascertain how well the entrance skin doses given in a particular department correlate with those shown in Table 4.2. To ensure confidence in the results of such measurements, the dosimeters should only be from a laboratory recognized as competent by a national regulatory body (e.g. the Health and Safety Executive in the UK). Suitably calibrated Thermo-luminescent dosimeters (TLDs) are available from medical physics departments or the NRPB in the UK (see appendix for addresses).

Table 4.3 gives details of mean organ doses, from some common X-ray examinations and Table 4.4 shows the mean and maximum doses. Tables 4.5 and 4.6 deal with skin and organ doses for children, and Table 4.8 with nuclear medicine examinations.

Table 4.1 EFFECTIVE DOSE EQUIVALENTS (IN mSv) OF COMMON EXAMIN-
ATIONS

	Mean	Minimum	Maximum
Lumbar spine			
Whole examination	2.15	0.37	7.37
AP only*	0.9	0.09	6.87
Lateral only*	0.53	0.07	3.14
L5–S1 lateral	0.50	0.05	2.06
Chest			
PA and lateral (1.3 films)	0.05	0.01	1.32
PA only	0.02	< 0.01	0.18
Lateral only	0.13	0.01	1.20
Skull			
Three views	0.15	0.01	0.50
AP only	0.06	0.01	0.21
Lateral only	0.03	0.01	0.13
Abdomen			
AP	1.39	0.12	9.94
Thoracic spine			
Two views	0.92	0.16	4.39
AP only	0.48	0.07	3.13
Lateral only	0.29	0.01	1.42
Pelvis	1.22	0.09	5.77
Intravenous urogram			
(8 films)	4.4	1.4	35
Barium meal			
(8 films; including average screening time)	3.8	0.6	24
Barium enema			
(8/9 films)	7.7	2.9	34
Cholecystography			
(4/5 films)	1	0.1	5

AP = Anteroposterior; PA = posteroanterior.
*There is a larger difference between the AP and lateral views due to the
variation in cassette sizes used for the AP view. The cassette size used for the
lateral view is 20 × 40 or 30 × 40 cm; the AP can be 35 × 43 cm.
Other source material used in Table 4.1 is as follows:
1. Personal communications from Paul Shrimpton and Barry Wall at NRPB
2. Nishizawa et al. (Jan. 1991) Determinations of organ doses and effective
   dose equivalents from computed tomographic examinations. *British Journal
   of Radiology* **64**
3. Guidance notes of The Arsac Secretariat, 1988.
4. Core of Knowledge course handbook, Hammersmith Hospital, Department
   of Physics and Diagnostic Radiology 1988.
5. Lotz et al. (1987). Low Dose Pelvimetry with Biplane Digital Radiography.
   Acta Radiologica **28**.

Table 4.2 ENTRANCE SKIN DOSES FROM COMMON EXAMINATIONS

Procedure	View	Dose (mGy)
Lumbar spine	AP	9.2(× 6)
	Lateral	23 (× 5)
	L5–S1	39 (× 3)
Chest	PA	0.2(× 6)
	Lateral	1.5(× 7)
Skull	PA	4.7(× 2)
	Lateral	2.2(× 2)
Abdomen	AP	8.4(× 7)
Thoracic spine	AP	6.5(× 3)
	Lateral	17 (× 3)
Pelvis	AP	6.6(× 5)
Fluoroscopy		0.3 mGy/min
(dose rate at skin surface		(× 1.3 for poor collimation;
under minimum dose rate		× 2 for large patient–
conditions)		intensifier distance;
		× 3 for high dose rate
		option selected;
		× 5 for magnified
		image – greater for
		combinations)

Figures in brackets are the factors by which the maximum doses exceeded the mean doses recorded in the NRPB survey. Far higher doses probably do occur, and may be justified in particular clinical situations. These figures give a guide to the range usually encountered. The skin doses quoted in this table are from the same report (NRPB R200) as the effective dose equivalents in Table 4.1. Knowledge of these skin doses can be used to approximate effective dose equivalents for each examination.

Skeletal survey

Add the effective dose equivalents together to give the total for the study, e.g. for myeloma the usual series would be: posteroanterior chest, lateral skull, anteroposterior and lateral lumbar and thoracic spines, pelvis to include the upper third of the femora. The effective dose equivalents are:

$$0.02 + 0.03 + 0.48 + 0.29 + 0.9 + 0.53 + 1.22 = 3.47 \, \text{mSv,}$$
assuming optimal technique

This compares favourably with a technetium 99m bone scan at 5.0 mSv. The bone scan may pick up metastases far earlier than plain radiography, and is less unpleasant for a patient in severe pain than a full set of radiographs.

Table 4.3 MEAN ORGAN DOSES FROM SOME COMMON X-RAY PROCEDURES

	Breast dose (mGy)	Red bone marrow dose (mGy)	Lung dose (mGy)	Thyroid dose (mGy)
Lumbar spine				
Complete exam	0.07(× 4)	1.4(× 4)	0.3(× 4)	< 0.01
AP only	0.04	0.2	0.14	< 0.01
Lateral only	0.01	0.5	0.10	< 0.01
Lateral L5–S1 only	< 0.01	0.6	0.01	< 0.01
Chest (conventional, not high kVp)				
PA projection	0.01(× 13)	0.02(× 10)	0.08(× 8)	0.01(× 6)
AP projection	0.2	0.01	0.07	0.06
Lateral projection	0.4	0.1	0.3	0.06
*Skull**				
3 views	< 0.01	0.15(× 4)	0.01(× 4)	0.39(× 4)
AP	< 0.01	0.07(× 3)	< 0.01	0.25(× 3)
PA	< 0.01	0.06(× 3)	< 0.01 (0.01)	0.09(× 2)
Lateral	< 0.01	0.03(× 4)	< 0.01	0.04(× 4)
Abdomen				
AP	0.02(× 9)	0.27(× 8)	0.06(× 7)	< 0.01
Thoracic spine				
AP	1.06(× 7)	0.22(× 7)	1.05(× 7)	1.15(× 7)
Lateral	0.06(× 6)	0.32(× 5)	1.32(× 5)	0.07(× 7)
Pelvis				
AP	< 0.01 (0.02)	0.16(× 5)	< 0.01 (0.02)	< 0.01
PA	< 0.01 (0.02)	0.27	< 0.01 (0.02)	< 0.01

AP = Anteroposterior; PA = posteroanterior.
*Eye doses are not available from the document, but the reduction in thyroid dose achieved by using PA rather than AP positioning will be mirrored if not bettered when eye doses are compared.
Figures in brackets are the factors by which the maximum doses exceeded the mean doses recorded in the NRPB survey and represent a worse-case scenario.

It must be noted that the effective dose equivalent varies from one model of computed tomography scanner to another and from manufacturer to manufacturer. In a 1990 paper (Shrimpton et al. of NRPB) the dose characteristics of four frequently used scanners were compared and found to be consistently lower for some and consistently higher for others. The image quality may

Table 4.4 MEAN (MAXIMUM) GONAD DOSES (mGy) FROM SOME COMMON EXAMINATIONS

Examination	Testes	Uterus	Ovary
Chest			
PA only	< 0.01	< 0.01	< 0.01
Lumbar spine			
AP	0.03 (0.29)	1.93 (14.89)	1.48 (11.58)
Lateral	0.01 (0.08)	0.48 (3.12)	0.97 (5.97)
L5–S1	0.01 (0.05)	0.62 (2.78)	1.41 (5.89)
Pelvis			
AP	4.29 (20.48)	1.55 (6.89)	1.14 (5.03)

AP = Anteroposterior; PA = posteroanterior.

Table 4.5 RADIATION SKIN DOSES FOR CHILDREN IN mGy

Projection/study	Lowest doses	Lowest : highest ratio
Skull AP/PA (also post nasal space)	0.030	× 43
Spine lateral	0.043	× 48
Abdomen AP	0.024	× 48
Thorax AP/PA	0.020	× 17
Pelvis (congenital dysplasia of the hips)	0.007	× 186
Premature chest (mobile unit)	0.017	× 27
Infant chest (mobile unit)	0.021	× 39

AP = Anteroposterior; PA = posteroanterior.
(ref: Fendel et al. British Institute of Radiology Report 20 1988)

of course vary, and the improved image quality offered in the higher-dose scanners may reduce the number of slices required so that the overall effective dose equivalent per examination is similar.

Nishizawa et al. in their paper of January 1991 in the BJR gave generally lower figures for effective dose equivalents for computed tomography scans, with a far smaller variation from manufacturer to manufacturer. There are several possible explanations:

1. The Japanese techniques are often different to those used in the UK, e.g. concerning regularity of contrast enhancement, and the use of different protocols.
2. The Japanese adult population is on average smaller in stature than those in the UK.

Table 4.6 ORGAN DOSES FOR CHILDREN IN mGy PER UNIT ENTRANCE DOSE IN mGy

	Skull AP	Skull lateral	Thorax AP	Thorax PA	Abdomen AP	Pelvis AP
Brain	0.285	0.351	0.003	0.003	< 0.0005	< 0.0005
Eye lenses	1.299	0.563	0.006	0.002	0.003	< 0.0005
Lungs	0.047	0.020	0.466	0.479	0.200	0.001
Ovaries	< 0.0005	< 0.0005	0.003	0.001	0.569	0.505
Testes	< 0.0005	< 0.0005	< 0.0005	< 0.0005	0.124	0.184
Thyroid	0.417	0.585	0.799	0.163	0.012	< 0.0005
Uterus	< 0.0005	< 0.0005	0.001	< 0.0005	0.627	0.636
Skeleton	0.694	0.691	0.351	0.502	0.449	0.306
Red bone marrow	0.078	0.066	0.042	0.061	0.075	0.057
Total body	0.123	0.122	0.126	0.136	0.235	0.134

AP = Anteroposterior; PA = posteroanterior.
Skeletal survey for non-accidental injury: six films: chest X-ray plus upper humeri, skull anteroposterior + lateral views, pelvis and upper femora, lower legs and ankles, mid-humerus to wrists. The whole child on one projection can give a 30% higher dose than separate coned views of each part. Diagnostic quality is far superior on coned projections. 'Babygrams' are to be discouraged.

Table 4.7 MEAN EFFECTIVE DOSE EQUIVALENTS (mSv) FOR COMPUTED TOMOGRAPHY SCANS

	UK data	Japanese data: mean (maximum)
Head	3.5	0.5 (0.692)
Chest	9.1	6.9 (14.05)
Abdomen	8.8	3.7 (7.3)
Lumbar spine	6.0	Not available
Pelvis	9.4	3.6 (6.17) male; 7.13 (12.53) female

Figures quoted are for standard technique. Doses for enhanced slices are ≃ 20% higher than for plain scans.

3. The use of local technology with similar designs may well have helped to restrict closely the variation in doses between one unit and another.
4. The paper concerned uses slightly different methods to calculate effective dose equivalents to those used in the UK.

Discussion

The effective dose equivalents are extremely high for computed tomography scan examinations compared to plain radiographic

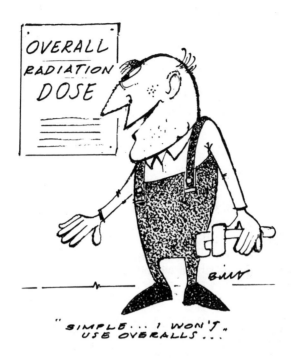

"SIMPLE... I WON'T USE OVERALLS..."

examinations, and this should be considered carefully when such scans are requested.

Pelvimetry

Scanogram. To replace conventional pelvimetry: ovary doses: 0.12 mGy. (1.7 mGy conventional technique pelvimetry.) (Lotz et al., 1987).

Mammography

Effective dose equivalent 0.35 mSv for full examination. (NRPB, *Medical Radiation 'At a glance'*).

Angiography

Techniques and imaging protocols vary from centre to centre and between radiologists at the same centre. To estimate doses, add the screening time dose (Table 4.2) to the dose for each projection (Table 4.1) to give an overall dose figure. When contrast is present within the patient, the exposure factors usually require a small increase to maintain film blackening. This corresponds to an increase in dose to the patient of up to 20% due to increased radiation absorption in the contrast medium.

Sample calculation

Transfemoral arteriogram:
2 min fluoroscopy: 0.6 mGy/min (a longer patient intensifier distance is required due to the sterile field) = 1.2 mGy.
For one run: skin dose for control film = 6.6 mGy.
two films of pelvis with contrast + (2 × 8) 16 mGy +
two films of knee with contrast + (2 × 4) 8 mGy +
five films of tibia and fibula with + (5 × 3) 25 mGy = 56.8 mGy entrance skin dose.

Organ doses can be estimated from the appropriate proportions of each of these radiographic projections.

These examinations can now be compared from a dosimetric viewpoint to those from digital subtraction angiography (below), and indirectly with those from computed tomography (Table 4.7).

Digital subtraction angiography (DSA) (B.I.R. Report 20 Taylor et al.)

The doses for this procedure are high, but it is less invasive than conventional angiography and thus the risks from other aspects of the examination are lower.

Entrance skin dose for conventional cardiac   200–400 mGy
catheterization
Entrance skin dose for DSA cardiac catheterization 300–800 mGy
For postoanterior abdominal examination:
   Intra-arterial contrast selected 0.7 mGy per test frame
                                      2.0 mGy per frame
   Intravenous contrast selected 3–5 mGy per frame

Table 4.8 NUCLEAR MEDICINE EXAMINATIONS (ALL FIGURES ARE FOR TECHNETIUM 99m STUDIES, UNLESS INDICATED)

	Mars serial number*	Maximum usual activity (MBq)	Effective dose equivalent (mSv)	Estimated uterus dose (mGy)
Thyroid imaging	(43.a.1.ii)	80	1.0	0.6
Brain imaging	(43.a.1.v)	500	7.0	4.0
Lung perfusion	(43.a.3.i)	100	1.0	0.3
Lung ventilation	(43.a.12)	80 (aerosol)	0.6	0.5
Bone imaging	(43.a.4.)	600	5.0	4.0
Liver imaging	(43.a.7.i)	80	1.0	0.2
Kidney DTPA	(43.a.5.i)	300	3.0	2.0
Kidney DMSA	(43.a.6)	80	1.0	0.4
Meckel's diverticulum	(43.a.1.iv)	400	5.0	3.0
Indium-labelled white blood cell	(49.a.3)	40	24.0	5.0
Gallium 67	(31.a.1) Tumour or abscess imaging	150	18.0	12.0

*Mars serial number refers to the examination serial number as defined by the Medical Administration of Radioactive Substances legislation. Administration of Radioactive Substances Advisory Committee licences are granted for specific examinations by serial number. Several different examinations, using different isotopes and/or doses, are available to image the same organ or system. Use of these specific serial numbers eliminates confusion (see also Chapter 12).
DTPA = Diethylenetriamine pentacetic acid; DMSA = Dimercapto-succinate.

The dose is higher during intravenous studies because the subject contrast is reduced, and more radiation is needed to produce the necessary image quality.

Mean effective dose equivalents: Carotid 4 mSv; Femoral 4 mSv; Hepatic 22 mSv; Renal 14 mSv (Steele and Temperton, 1992).

Discussion

It is relatively easy to carry on with long screening times and extra projections during DSA. The contrast volumes and concentration used do not limit the investigation as they do with conventional angiography.

DSA is very much at the higher end of the dose range in diagnostic radiology. This modality has definite patient benefits in terms of procedure safety and acceptability, but it is not necessarily a radiation dose reduction technique.

5

Quality assurance in the X-ray department

Many aspects of the X-ray department and its personnel contribute to the final standard of the radiographic examination and patient satisfaction. Output, processor and other equipment tests are an important factor, but are not the only contributors to the final product. The radiation protection adviser has an essential advisory role in the design and implementation of a quality assurance programme. He or she should be consulted on all aspects of this, from the frequency of measurements to the tolerances allowed.

A patient arrives at the X-ray reception desk, and hands in a *request form*. Are adequate patient and clinical details included on the request form? Is the correct anatomical site or examination requested? Is the form legally complete?

What happens to it next? Ideally it is checked out by a competent radiographer or radiologist.

Is the *administrative back-up system* quick and efficient? (A computer system is often of great assistance.) Are previous films available when and where required?

How long does the patient wait? Are waiting conditions pleasant, comfortable and warm? (Comfortable patients are usually more co-operative during their X-ray examination.) Is there a separate waiting corner for children with toys, crayons and posters?

Devise a patient satisfaction questionnaire. Encourage the consumer to suggest improvements.

Departmental protocol

When the examination takes place, are the correct projections or views taken? Does the department have a standard protocol

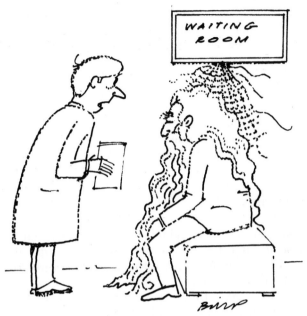

"SO SORRY TO KEEP YOU WAITING SIR, WE HAVE
BEEN DOING OUR QUALITY ASSURANCE CHECKS."

handbook? If not, why not? (Such a handbook can be extremely
useful in reducing unnecessary radiographs, saving patient dose,
time and resources.) Is gonad protection always applied to
children and adults? (Refer to Patient dose reduction in diagnostic
radiology – NRPB, Vol. 1, NO. 3. 1990.)

Processor quality control

Are the processors functioning reliably? The problems of variable
processor results with modern microprocessor-controlled units,
automixers and automatic film handling are far less frequent
now than they were in the past. Climate conditions can have
an effect, but generally processor quality assurance may seem
to be a waste of effort. If this arises in your department, a possible
option is to perform processor quality assurance as an occasional
project. It can be run by a new member of staff for a limited

period, possibly in conjunction with a reject analysis programme.

It is extremely important, however, to have regular data on average film density and contrast, so that swift diagnosis is possible if a processing fault is suspected. Processing chemicals can arrive incorrectly labelled, replenishment pumps can fail, and airlocks can occur in pipework. None of these would be considered operator error, but all could have detrimental effects on film quality. Processor quality assurance is of far greater importance for mammography, 100/105 mm films, cathode ray tube and any other single-emulsion film, where less latitude exists before the image quality is rendered undiagnostic.

Reject analysis

This can be an extremely valuable tool. There are many excellent books on the subject and it would be of no value to rewrite them here. Particularly noteworthy is the British Institute of Radiology handbook, *Assurance of Quality in the Diagnostic X-ray Department*, published in 1988. Junior personnel may perceive a reject analysis programme as a witch-hunt. In order to gain the co-operation of all staff, it is advantageous to involve as many as practical in the project, from all grades, and to stress the positive outcomes.

The programme may reveal equipment problems, but it is unlikely that these were unknown previously. The identification of a particular area of poor technique or even an individual whose radiographic abilities require improvement is a problem which demands the utmost skill in its resolution. It is well worth holding regular update meetings between the reject analysis team and the other junior staff, to exchange ideas and to allow those who know they have technique problems to voice their own suggestions as to how to remedy them. This will give a more positive outlook to the entire project.

In-service training

Training sessions, possibly involving the help of outside experts (from a local radiography school, orthopaedic or paediatric hospital) are not only valuable aids in improving technique problems but often act as morale-boosting sessions for staff keen to progress with their careers. Exchanges between general and specialist hospitals can also be another low-cost method of getting the results required. Staff are loaned on an honorary contract basis between hospitals to help each other raise standards.

Equipment for quality assurance

The investment required for a well-equipped quality assurance programme runs to a sizeable capital sum. It is inadvisable to launch into such a programme from scratch, especially if no one in the department is trained in quality assurance. Regular courses are available; one person should be kept updated.

Digital radiation output meter

As a start, a digital radiation output meter (such as the Radcheck from Victoreen, USA) with an ionization chamber detector is ideal. There are a number of useful tests that can be performed with such a meter (output variation with timer, mA and kVp^2, for example) and this provides a pass/fail test as to whether X-rays are being produced on a suspected faulty unit.

The output meter can also be used to check reliability and linearity of timer stations, to verify increasing output with increasing mA, ensuring that the mA compensator is functioning. It may also be used for setting up exposure charts for new equipment. Ideally output is checked weekly and certainly before and after engineer visits, to ensure that output has not altered dramatically.

The real value of equipment quality assurance is in the investigation of apparent faults before booking an engineer. Sometimes the fault is disproved, saving on an engineer call-out. More often than not, the nature of the problem is ascertained and the engineer, when called, is alerted to it, does not waste expensive call-out time identifying the problem, and brings the correct test equipment and spares along to the site.

Junior radiographers may be extremely wary about reporting a fault to the superintendent, only to discover that it was a technique error or other operator fault. They then feel responsible for the costly engineer call-out. If these personnel are given the opportunity to diagnose and verify the fault, using in-house test equipment, either individually or in consultation with the quality assurance radiographer, the whole mood changes. Reporting suspected faults takes on a far less threatening aspect, faults are reported earlier and fewer repeats result from them.

The radiologist

However perfect the radiograph, the end result of a radiographic examination is the radiologist's report. That person's vision, concentration and pattern recognition abilities are the final factor in the quality chain. Stress, poor viewing-room conditions, frequent interruptions, overwork, long rota duties, eye strain and inaccurate visual correction can all have serious detrimental effects on the outcome. Regular eye-testing, healthy lifestyle and attention to working conditions all help to ensure optimum skill levels in these key members of the team.

Poor-quality radiographs prevent the optimum use of the radiologist's skills. He or she may be distracted from pathology by artefacts, film handling faults and other errors. Scribbled felt-tip pens replacing right and left markers are an example.

Poor positioning, incorrect exposure and inappropriate centring may distort anatomy and hide pathology.

The radiographer

The satisfaction for the radiographer in producing a technically superior radiograph can be enhanced by the knowledge that this film is more likely to yield an accurate diagnosis for the patient than an inferior one. Encouragement of high standards can reap great benefits for all staff. Radiographers should always see their own work *before* the patient leaves the department. This ensures job satisfaction as well as maintaining standards. Stress, overwork and uneven allocation of rota duties can all undermine radiographic performance.

Quality assurance

The time taken to carry out quality assurance is a sound investment – without it, we are using our patients as test phantoms. Patients come in all shapes and sizes, thus the over- or underexposed film may be due to misjudging the patient rather than an equipment fault.

Automatic exposure devices (AEDs) in some ways help to standardize results, but they can themselves malfunction. If they fail, they become unsafe. If the AED is positioned over an inappropriate area, it can give a poor result. The film is then repeated and may be no more diagnostic the second time, if the positioning is not amended. In some countries (Germany, for example), the AED chamber position is marked on the finished radiograph with a semi-opaque symbol. This confirms the AED chamber position, and helps identify incorrect positioning. AEDs can be successfully tested with a bucket of water and a cassette (see appendix to this chapter).

Dental X-rays

Dental X-ray units should not be forgotten. They operate at fixed kVp and mA, the only variable being the timer. However, collimation can be outside of the specification, causing irradiation of a larger area than necessary on every examination for which it is used. This reduces radiographic quality (due to extra scattered radiation) as well as increasing the radiation dose. The usual maximum field size for dental units in the UK is 6.0 cm (never more than 7.5 cm) diameter. Occasionally, units have been found irradiating an area of up to 12.0 cm diameter, giving an unnecessary eye and bone marrow dose to children and adults alike.

Collimation can be checked using an occlusal film or an ordinary X-ray cassette (see appendix to this chapter).

Fluoroscopy equipment

The Leeds TOR. TVF. test phantom is a particularly well-designed fluoroscopy test phantom. The dose rate can be checked using the digital output meter discussed earlier, but failing this, a rough guide to dose rate is available by observing the screening mA value (where such a meter is fitted) for a known thickness of phantom.

Coincidence of X-ray field and image intensifier input face should also be regularly checked using an ordinary cassette (see appendix to this chapter).

Kilovoltage

Much information is available from digital output meter measurements. At a given mA value the intensity of the radiation beam is proportional to $(kV)^2$. By plotting output against peak kilovoltage squared $(kV_p)^2$ (or square root of output against kV_p) the graph should plot as a straight line. If it does not, one suspects kV_p compensation error.

Filtration

At known kV_p values, the half-value thickness for aluminium can be translated into an approximate value for total filtration. At $80 \, kV_p$ the half-value thickness and total filtration are approximately equal. Provided $80 \, kV_p$ is verifiable, the filtration can be checked using the output meter and a set of pure aluminium filters. Ordinary sheet aluminium alloy is not suitable for this purpose; it must be pure to at least 99.9%, since most alloys contain copper to harden the aluminium, giving distorted results.

Computed tomography scanners (CT)

These should not be overlooked. Seek advice from the regional physics department or local equivalent, and the manufacturer. Regular imaging of a phantom should be carried out. The emphasis is on information content per unit of X-ray exposure, slice width, percentage noise and resolution.

Full evaluation of a CT unit requires the following phantoms:

1. A circular phantom of 320 mm external diameter, filled with water or water equivalent; the outer wall is of methyl methacrylate (Perspex).

2. A circular phantom of 200 mm outer diameter, to include an outer 5 mm of bone substitute material, filled with water or water equivalent material.

3. An anatomically shaped phantom (similar in cross-section to the adult human abdomen), filled with water or water-equivalent material, with low-contrast detection objects, a large air hole, and a large hole for inserts of various types, such as an air-bone edge.

See Bibliography for further reading.

Appendix

Many useful quality assurance tests can be performed without the need for special equipment.

Automatic exposure devices

Place a water-filled bucket over the chamber. Expose the film and process. Compare it with other chambers and previous results. Carry out sensitometry at the same time to exclude processor variations.

Dental set collimation

Using a ballpoint pen, make a cross in the centre of an occlusal film. Expose the film to the beam at the usual focus to film distance, centring it to the cross. Process and examine. Diameter should not exceed 6.0 cm, and must not exceed 7.5 cm. This will be apparent from the occlusal film. If an occlusal film is not available, mount four intraoral films, overlap and mark, so that they can be reassembled. Expose and process. Examine after reassembly.

The patient

Quality assurance has been written about at length – there are now a large number of excellent publications available. However, the ultimate end user of the radiographic service is the patient, whose view of quality is based on length of waiting time, the professionalism and pleasantness of the receptionist and radiographer, the standard of waiting area provided, the provision of reading materials and information about likely delays. Time spent caring for patients waiting, and indeed keeping them informed, is every bit as important as performing quality checks on the equipment.

Tomography

The path can be traced using a piece of lead with a hole in the centre, supported between the table top and fulcrum level. Make a perpendicular beam exposure, and then expose with tomographic movement. The resultant film will show a line with a spot, ideally in the centre of the line, which should be of uniform density. Any departure from these two conditions indicates a malfunction.

Another useful check is the fan test. This is carried out using a cassette, supported vertically within a syringe box, among the syringes, with the shorter edge parallel to the beam path. The name marker must be placed at the bottom. The resultant image is of a fan-shaped area. The angle is equal to the exposure angle.

Legends

Barium sulphate powder can be used very effectively to prepare home-made legends and numbers, using auto repair resin, or epoxy resin glue as a hardening agent.

Testing coincidence of fluoroscopy beam and explorator

Use a 35 × 43 cm cassette in the cassette slot. Attach a radiopaque object to the centre of the field, open the collimators fully and position the explorator as far from the X-ray tube as possible. Screen for 10 seconds and develop the film. The opaque object should appear in the centre of the image and the blackened area should not be larger than the intensifier face.

Major tests to be performed and frequency recommended

1. Output in mGy per mAs – weekly. At different mA settings – monthly. At different kV settings – monthly (ionization chamber output meter).
2. Kilovoltage accuracy – monthly, at all regularly used mA stations, to verify correct operation of mA compensator (kV meter or penetrameter cassette).
3. Fluoroscopy dose rate – weekly (ionization chamber).
4. Fluoroscopy resolution and contrast threshold – weekly (TOR. TVF. phantom).
5. Fluoroscopy beam coincidence with image intensifier using a cassette – quarterly.
6. Processor performance – weekly or twice weekly (sensitometer and densitometer). More frequently for mammography; twice daily for mammography screening. Daily if using regeneration on developer solution.
7. Timer accuracy and reproducibility – monthly (timer test tool or output ionization chamber if no timer test tool is available).
8. Filtration – quarterly (pure aluminium filters and ionization chamber).
9. Collimation and beam alignment – quarterly on most units. Monthly on mobile unit used on special care baby unit. Possibly required monthly on tomography equipment. Mechanical shock to these units in use can cause misalignment of the collimator (collimation test tool and beam alignment tool; also possible with paper clips. The proper tool is taken more seriously by the engineer).
10. Tomography performance – quarterly (tomography test tool: several are commercially available. Check with other users before purchase as some are designed to look pretty rather than provide the required information).
11. Electrical and mechanical safety checks – at every use. Do a more thorough inspection monthly. *This can save a life.*
12. Image resolution – annually (star or bar test pattern). More frequently on equipment used for macroradiography.
13. Automatic exposure devices – monthly (phantom and film in cassette).
14. Screens and cassettes: film screen contact and sensitivity –

annually and additionally if a cassette has been dropped. Use film screen contact test tool and TOR rad test tool. Sensitometric exposure on the film used for sensitivity check will exclude processor variation. Check sensitivity against a new screen of same type, but beware of film variations.
15. Darkroom and film storage – quarterly.
16. Film illuminators and viewing room conditions – quarterly. Large illuminator variations will cause film acceptability problems around the hospital and even around the department.

6
Dose reduction and gonad protection

Introduction

Whilst the population dose from diagnostic radiology is a small fraction of the total (which includes background and cosmic radiation), there is no doubt that it is the largest manmade and therefore controllable part of the dose received. Any economically and socially acceptable means of reducing that dose, without compromising the diagnostic value of the procedure, must be worth implementing. Fortunately the dose reduction changes which have the greatest potential for lowering patient doses are also those with the lowest – sometimes zero – cost implications, and in a few instances actually save money. The main factors which can reduce patient doses are as follows:

1. Don't irradiate the patient at all: exclude non-essential studies and/or substitute ionizing radiation with ultrasound, magnetic resonance imaging (MRI) and endoscopy.
2. Modify the procedure so that fewer radiographs or shorter screening (fluoroscopy) times are required. Vet carefully higher dose requests.
3. Use the most sensitive imaging method consistent with the minimum necessary image quality, e.g. superfast screens and film, photofluorography instead of radiography.
4. Use the smallest possible field size, as well as postcollimation and gonad protection.
5. Use the least possible attenuation between patient and image receptor. Modify the beam spectrum (filtration) to optimize this parameter.
6. Use the greatest possible focus to skin distance.

Radiation dose reduction strategies will mostly fall into one of these six categories. Clearly the greatest dose reduction opportunities lie in avoiding the examination in the first instance.

As members of the radiographic and radiological professions, we are honour-bound to act in such a way as to minimize the risk of genetic damage to our patients, however low the probability of such damage.

So much to do – where do we start?

A vast range of dose reduction and limitation options is available to the imaging department. Sadly, unlimited resources are not available for these changes, and thus they cannot all be carried out at once. Faced with these realities, the busy imaging department manager may feel unable to act because the finance is not available to put them all into action immediately.

An excellent booklet prepared by the NRPB/RCR in the UK, 'Patient dose reduction in diagnostic radiology', details the savings possible for the various options. The first priority must be to eliminate clinically unhelpful examinations and reduce repeat rates, reduce numbers of films per examination, and reduce fluoroscopy times. These measures together offer a potential saving of 5800 man Sv. Clinical audit in conjunction with the radiologists has a key role in this area.

An additional strategy which could further reduce hospital mean doses by 1300 man Sv involves the use of new technology such as carbon fibre components, faster film–screen combinations, rare earth filtration, and constant potential waveform generators, all of which require extra investment. Use of additional rare earth filtration requires an increase in exposure factors. This may accelerate wear on the tube and demand longer exposure times, increasing the possibility of movement unsharpness.

The advantages of opting for the first priority, as described above, are as follows:

1. There is no requirement to invest heavily in extra equipment or equipment modifications.

2. Fewer films per patient results in savings to the departmental budget on film and processing chemicals, and reduced time spent per patient on radiography and radiological reporting.
3. Fewer films per patient means less space is required to store films.
4. Fewer films and shorter fluoroscopy times mean either less wear and tear on equipment or increased patient throughput and shorter waiting lists, with a real potential for a better service to patients.
5. Dose reduction *per patient* to radiology/radiography staff.

If the approach taken is to reduce films and fluoroscopy times, reduce repeat rates, and eliminate clinically unhelpful examinations, when everything possible has been achieved here the savings made can be used to finance the capital investments such as replacing constant potential generators, carbon fibre components, rare earth filters and new superfast intensifying screens. To concentrate all our efforts on making every examination the lowest dose procedure possible is not necessarily ideal. This is especially true if a proportion of those examinations should either not take place at all or could be as diagnostically useful with half the number of films.

An analogy would be to invest heavily in measures to reduce the pain experienced during dental treatment, but not to improve the accuracy of the diagnosis. Many unnecessary fillings would take place, but the patients would not suffer greatly during drilling.

Methods and techniques for dose reduction

The development of new techniques and materials for use within medical imaging has brought enormous potential for dose reduction. Their universal speedy adoption has been delayed by a variety of factors – practical, financial and social – which shall be discussed in turn. Some of the scientific breakthroughs have dramatic dose-saving potential, but only in limited applications. These should be adopted as soon as possible, particularly where the radiography of children is involved.

Substitution of non-ionizing investigations

Replacement of one diagnostic investigation by another is a matter for clinical judgement by a radiologist. Examples are ultrasound and digestive system endoscopy and pressure investigations (in irritable bowel disease).

In the modern climate of value for money, replacing an ionizing radiation investigation for a non-ionizing radiation procedure, which is often more acceptable to the patient for other reasons, is a definite improvement in the service provided. These points are well worth making to purchasing health authorities at the contracting stage.

Advances in imaging practice have in many instances offered an alternative to ionizing radiation investigations. An additional benefit to the patient may be that there is usually then no need to use iodinated contrast media, which carries a small but appreciable mortality risk. Three such examples are in the investigation of urinary tract infections in young women, in studies of lower lumbar spine neurological symptoms and in the investigation of colonic problems.

Pelvic and renal ultrasound and a plain abdominal radiograph were found to give more useful information than an intravenous urogram (IVU) (BJR March 1991). Several important findings were apparent on ultrasound such as renal abscess, ectopic pregnancy and fibroids which were not apparent on IVU. If these patients had had an IVU alone (with its risks of side-effects, mortality and high cost) these important clinical abnormalities might have gone undetected.

Prior to the introduction of MRI, patients presenting with low back pain and neurological symptoms would undergo myelography. Postprocedural complications are not unusual, admission to hospital is usually necessary and the procedure is thoroughly unpleasant for the patient. MRI is an outpatient procedure, no medication is required, it is not unpleasant, and the most likely complication is the accidental cancellation of a credit card by the magnetic field.

The investigation of irritable bowel syndrome using pressure studies, and the use of colonoscopy for query colitis and polyps are both non-ionizing radiation investigations replacing barium enema, which is a very high-dose study.

Exclusion of non-essential views

Non-essential views should be excluded from the routine for referrals to the department. Preparation of a departmental radiographic protocol handbook is a useful way forward here.

Dose reduction technique modifications

Modifications such as the use of non-grid techniques, e.g. ultrafine collimation and air-gap technique should be made. Focus to patient distances should be increased. Beam-shaping filters should be used for barium enemas, hilar tomography and other examinations where different patient thicknesses are examined in one exposure.

New technology

1. Constant potential generators can be used to improve the composition of the X-ray beam. A beam containing a greater proportion of high-energy photons is produced, giving less skin dose for the same imaging information.
2. Superfast rare earth intensifying screens minimize radiation doses. Optical sensitizers increase film–screen combination speed.
3. Modified filtration materials such as erbium, yttrium, copper or increased thicknesses of aluminium increase the proportion of image-forming photons in the beam. Also in mammography.
4. Carbon fibre (which has a low atomic number) cassette fronts, table tops and grid interspacings help reduce radiation dose.

Dose limitation

1. Limit the radiographic views taken, especially during complex examinations such as barium enema or meal, and IVU.
2. Limit fluoroscopy time to the minimum commensurate with good diagnostic results.
3. Iris collimators for fluoroscopy tubes reduce unnecessary irradiation as the image intensifier input face is circular rather than square.

Training

Better training in radiation protection for radiologists and radiographers (both pre- and postqualification), related to an ongoing reject analysis programme, means that fewer repeat radiographs are necessary. The ultimate aim is that every exposure is useful.

Dose reduction strategy

A dose reduction strategy working party can be established within the department (as suggested by UK Health Department Circular H.C.(89)18 and The Healing Arts Radiation Protection Guidelines; Ontario, Canada). This body should constantly monitor radiation doses, and have the power to fund changes or enforce modifications to existing practice. Membership could include the quality assurance radiographer, paediatric X-ray specialist, radiography manager, senior radiologist and radiation protection adviser. Apart from impressing government inspectors, it is a platform where dose reduction techniques and measures can be discussed. The minutes of such meetings can be used as evidence that the issue is seriously considered in the department.

Quality assurance (see also Chapter 5)

A comprehensive quality assurance programme should be established, monitoring especially criteria which affect radiation dose, such as collimation.

Computed tomography (CT) – supervision

The relatively high doses given in CT compared to conventional radiography should be widely publicized throughout the medical and dental professions. CT should only be carried out with the approval of a senior radiologist, only used where appropriate and in conjunction with the correct diagnostic work-up to suit each case. The details of the examination must be tailored so that the best possible diagnostic information is available, but no more slices than necessary are performed. Technique can be modified to reduce markedly the dose to critical organs (such as the eye during CT of the head). These techniques may be no more costly than angling the gantry or the patient's head during the scan so that the beam does not pass straight through the eyes.

Examinations only where outcome affects patient treatment

Patients should be referred for examinations only where it will affect the treatment. Many radiological examinations are extremely unpleasant for the patient and this alone is a justification for performing them only where prognosis will benefit.

Use of national guidance on dose reduction

National guidance on dose reduction should be adopted rapidly. In the UK: the National Radiological Protection Board document Patient dose reduction in diagnostic radiology and the Royal College of Radiologists' handbook *Making The Best Use of a Department of Radiology* are two such publications. The radiologist's role as the imaging expert within the hospital should be accepted more generally.

Health screening

Where no family history of breast carcinoma exists, mammography breast screening should only be performed on women over 50 years of age. Below this age, the number of cancers induced by the radiation used may exceed the numbers diagnosed, and an overall detriment rather than benefit will result. The attempts by some private health care providers to revise this limit downwards should be discouraged. Employment radiographic screening must be properly justified, and should be included as part of the occupational exposure of the worker (Calverd, BIR Report 20 1989, undocumented).

Radiography in pregnancy

No pregnant women should be X-rayed to assess fetal development unless ultrasound is not available. Low-dose techniques should be used for pelvimetry, i.e. superfast rare earth intensifying screens and carbon fibre components or, where possible, digital scanography using a CT scanner (see Chapter 7).

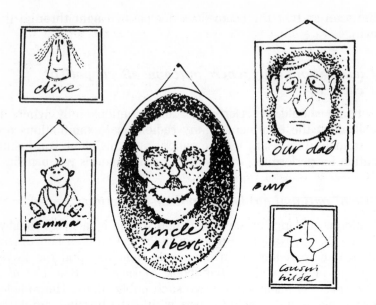

Availability of previous radiographs

Serious measures must be taken to improve the availability of previous films. Computerized radiology systems are helpful, but generally, there is a lack of interest in restoring radiographs to their correct resting place, that results in the repetition of large numbers of radiographs in every hospital every year.

In the private sector in the UK and certain other countries, patients retain their own films. This tends to be extremely successful until the person moves house.

The problem of missing radiographs wastes vast amounts of time and resources and causes endless frustration for all involved. There is a need for serious research into the problem and real progress to be made.

Use of clinical budgeting may help to control this problem, by giving a financial incentive to other hospital departments to co-operate in the return of radiographs.

Filmless radiography

Ultimately, the development of the filmless imaging department will enable all radiographic images to be stored on a computer system. At the time of writing, the number of megabytes required digitally to archive one examination was not dissimilar to the entire memory store of an average-sized personal computer. As technology progresses, the cost of such storage will fall rapidly and the filmless department will become a practical proposition.

Radiographs will never leave the department, but will be viewed on a terminal on the ward, in the clinic or at the general practice surgery.

Reduction in non-essential radiography/radiology

This list is taken from the joint NRPB and Royal College of Radiology publication 'Patient dose reduction in diagnostic radiology' with some extra comments from a consultant radiologist.

Non-essential views to be withdrawn from the *routine* projections list include:

- Submentovertical skull.
- Coned lateral pituitary fossa.
- Occipitofrontal – OF – and lateral sinuses (only occipitomental – OM – is required).
- Cervical spine flexion/extension (except in preoperative rheumatoid patients with anaesthetic risk) and oblique views.
- Odontoid peg should only be done in trauma (and possibly in congenital problems).
- Lateral chest.
- Erect abdomen.
- In lumbar spine coned L5–S1 and sacroiliac joints, obliques.
- In urinary tract: ultrasound is always the first-line investigation. IVU 1-min film, postmicturition film and more than six films.
- Cholecystogram: more than four films; ultrasound should always be the first-line investigation.
- Barium enema: postevacuation film.
- Knee: skyline and tunnel (anteroposterior and lateral only as routine).

Abandoning a small number of clinically unhelpful radiographs has a dual benefit – saving radiation dose to the patient (and staff), and reducing wastage of resources, which can be redirected towards cutting waiting lists and improving facilities.

Exclusion of non-essential views

One method of reducing the number of unnecessary radiographs is the preparation of an official X-ray department handbook. Other departments such as orthopaedics, rheumatology, trauma and paediatrics must be consulted in the preparation of this useful document. The resultant booklet will help ensure that the correct views are taken, and that unnecessary views are not. This is a valuable aid for new staff joining from another hospital. Arguments by a radiographer about not producing extra views are sometimes perceived by referring clinicians as laziness or lack of co-operation. Far from the case, it is very much easier for the radiographer to press on and produce the extra views, but the higher aim of dose limitation is then neglected, precious resources may be wasted – all with serious implications for the morale of the personnel involved. The publication of handbooks of departmental X-ray routine, along with clear guidance for when these recommendations should be disregarded, can be considered a priority for the proper management of X-ray services.

Gonad protection

Whenever the area of interest is not immediately under or adjacent to the gonads, it is in every way beneficial to employ gonad shielding or protection. The valuable public relations benefit of gonad shielding should not be overlooked. Using this equipment makes a statement to our patients – 'I have considered your safety and taken these measures to protect you and your future generations'.

Dirty, torn or tatty gonad shields do not make such a statement. They should be cleaned, repaired or replaced where appropriate.

Results of a 1991 Consumers Association report in the UK indicated high levels of patient dissatisfaction if gonad protection is not used.

Gonad protection may be used on all patients regardless of age or childbearing capacity. The benefits of such a policy are as follows:

1. Practice makes perfect. Currently, gonad shielding is used only on the minority of patients where it is of great importance and occasional errors are thus more likely.
2. If a gonad shield is incorrectly positioned on an elderly patient, and a repeat becomes necessary, the patient does not suffer genetic damage.
3. If gonad protection is a habit, it is far less likely to be forgotten in the cases where it is vital. It should not be overlooked that many women can and do become pregnant in their 40s. For men there is no upper limit.
4. If referring clinicians become accustomed to seeing gonad shielding on every film, in a case where it is likely to mask important information they will indicate the fact on the request form and signal '*Please do not use gonad shielding*'.

The fact that gonad shielding has been used should be indicated on the request form by the radiographer. If the case is later subject to a coexisting pregnancy investigation, such an indication is valuable protection for the personnel involved.

The male patient

Gonad protection for the male patient most often involves collimating the testes out of the beam altogether. Additional lead shielding (to reduce any contribution from extrafocal and scattered radiation) may also be required. Many well-designed devices are available commercially.

It is also beneficial to ask the patient to pull down his underpants. This allows the testes to drop away from the body and further reduce any radiation to them. This measure is especially important with the modern style of briefs which support the testes well up on to the pubic bone.

The female patient

It is statistically likely that 20% of women of childbearing capacity between the ages of 18 and 30 are pregnant at any one time. This figure is considerably higher than birth data because it includes women who miscarry or undergo terminations.

In the non-pregnant female patient of childbearing capacity, the critical organ is the ovary. If one were to examine a diagram showing the position of the ovaries in a number of women and girls, it would resemble the holes in a dartboard after a group of schoolboys had been busy playing. How then can we protect our patients from irradiation of the ovaries, if we cannot predict the position of these organs? The answer to this problem is twofold:

1. The probability of locating the ovaries is greatest in the area 2.5 cm medial to the anterior superior iliac spines.
2. Any measure to reduce the total amount of radiation incident upon the pelvic cavity will reduce internal scatter and in turn reduce the dose to the ovaries, even if they have not been accurately shielded.

Gonad shields are available commercially for female patients. However, the problem of equipment mysteriously disappearing from the X-ray department is observed in every hospital, and the use of lead rubber hand-made gonad shields is often a more cost-effective option. The shape and size can be determined by using the pelvic cavity image direct from a radiograph. Alternative types of gonad shield, such as magnetic mountings on to the front of the light beam diaphragm, are an elegant and practical arrangement. However unless these are pointed out to the patient, their public relations and patient satisfaction advantage is lost. Also, they can be misplaced and are no use where the gonads lie just outside the field. One is required for every room. A cheaper alternative is to use tiny, home-produced shapes mounted on the light beam diaphragm with self-adhesive putty or tape.

The 10-day and 28-day rules

The details of these policies are covered in Chapter 7.

The 10-day rule was introduced to reduce the probability of irradiation of an undiagnosed pregnancy. Female patients of childbearing capacity undergoing X-ray studies were only examined within the first 10 days following the onset of menstruation.

The 10-day rule has now been largely abandoned in favour of the 28-day rule. This is because there is no evidence for radiosensitivity of the conceptus in the first 4 weeks following the last menstrual period (LMP) (Wall, personal communication).

Consequently there is thought to be no particular benefit to the patient in restricting X-ray examinations only to the first 10 days after the LMP. Instead they can be allowed, without increased risk to the fetus, during the whole 28 days post LMP.

The aim of this change is to make life easier and less restrictive for the staff in busy X-ray departments. Generally, this change has been helpful. However, practical experience has shown this sometimes to be far from the case. Female patients are quite agreeable to discuss their menstrual history with X-ray receptionists, but the line of questioning now required under the 28-day rule protocol: 'Are you or might you be pregnant?' is of a very much more personal and intrusive nature. Such questioning via an interpreter can be fraught!

Additionally, patients X-rayed between 10 and 28 days post LMP who later found themselves to be pregnant suffer great anxiety about possible fetal damage, despite the efforts of dedicated radiologists and other clinicians to counsel them to the contrary. Women are well conversant with the idea that conception occurs at or about 14 days post LMP. The knowledge that the already developing fetus has undergone a dose of radiation is far more worrying to a patient than the same dose delivered to the unfertilized egg, even if it later becomes fertilized. For this reason, many X-ray departments have retained the 10-day rule, and found it to be advantageous.

90-day rule for male patients

Some recent publications have suggested that for male patients, especially those undergoing high-dose procedures such as barium enema, CT, IVU and pelvis studies, contraception should be used for the 3 months following the X-ray examination to avoid a radiation-damaged spermatozoon effecting a pregnancy with their partner. Such recommendations are not based on firm radiobiological evidence, and may cause great anxiety in our patients. It is not necessary to make such a recommendation, which could increase non-arrivals for examination!

Breast protection

The breast is an extremely radiosensitive organ, and is seldom protected during routine radiography, even where it lies near the field of interest. The radiosensitivity is greatest at puberty when the glandular tissue is growing rapidly. Carcinoma of the breast is a major cause of death in the developed world. It is therefore vital that every effort is made to avoid radiation-induced cancers adding to those statistics, however unlikely at the radiation levels under consideration. Examinations where the breast lies very near to the X-ray field, and should be shielded, include studies of humerus, IVU, abdomen and thoracic spine. Lead rubber shielding should be used to protect the breasts from scattered radiation, extrafocal radiation and inaccurate collimation in all such cases performed on female patients. A scoliosis shawl is now available to protect the breasts and lungs of young women during spinal studies.

Use of superfast rare earth intensifying screens

Television phosphors developed during the US space programme were a precursor to rare earth intensifying screens, which are now an integral part of the X-ray department's equipment. The reasons for their vastly increased efficiency over that for calcium tungstate are as follows. The higher atomic number of rare earth phosphors means that the absorption edge is in the right place and the conversion efficiency is higher, extending the response to higher energy photons. This allows the use of higher kV_p settings and increased filtration, which serves to reduce skin dose. The excellent efficiency of the phosphors allows the screens to be thinner than an equivalent calcium tungstate, improving resolution and contrast.

The green emitting phosphors which became available later allowed film manufacturers to exploit the advances in conventional photographic emulsion technology. This gives an overall improvement in film–screen combination sensitivity, with consequent dose savings.

The upper limit of film–screen speed is no longer set by resolution or contrast capabilities (both of which are excellent), but by the sensitivity of the imaging system itself. The grainy appearance (quantum mottle) on very fast films used with very fast screens is due to the small number of photons producing the image. (Raindrops appear as separate dots on the pavement when the rain firstarts to fall, but disappear when the rain is heavier, as they all join together.)

Where high resolution is not required, for example in scoliosis studies of the spine, the clinician can tolerate poor resolution and gain adequate information even with quantum mottle present, allowing extremely fast film–screen combinations to be used.

When first introduced, rare earth screens suffered a loss in speed over a period of 12–18 months and required replacement after 2 years. The stability of the phosphor materials is now excellent (a recent survey of 3-year-old screens showed no speed or resolution difference compared with a newly manufactured set from the same manufacturer, and of the same specification). Compared with traditional calcium tungstate screens, rare earths offer a speed advantage of double or better.

The transition between old and new screens in a department is made very much smoother if, using a radiation output meter, a phantom and the existing technique exposure chart, a new chart can be generated to remove the fear of the unknown and ensure successful results from the outset.

Modified filtration materials

All diagnostic X-ray tubes are required to have a minimum of 2.5 mm aluminium equivalent if operating above $70 \, kV_p$ (mammography tubes are excepted). Much has been written of the advantages of additional beam filtration to remove the 'soft' non-image-forming X-ray photons from the beam. There are however several provisos:

1. Gadolinium filters may have problems with their chemical stability – they have been known to oxidize and need replacing after a very short period.
2. The skin dose may be reduced, but organ doses and effective dose equivalents are not appreciably improved. Large increases in radiographic exposure time and milliamperage are required, increasing the probability of repeats due to movement unsharpness with the longer exposure times. (Shrimpton et al., 1988).
3. A filter is required on all X-ray tubes in the department. This involves heavy investment.

4. Contrast is reduced due to the higher average photon energy. This is not useful in paediatrics, orthopaedics or trauma radiography, where soft tissue detail is important.
5. The overall beam intensity is reduced, and consequently exposure time must be considerably increased (sometimes doubled or more), with resulting movement artefacts, especially in paediatrics, and involuntary movements in the cardiovascular system and gut.

Advantages

There are however advantages in specific applications, e.g. barium enema, where the subject contrast is very high (Unsworth, 1988) that erbium filters can be used to reduce dose without appreciable loss of image quality. Additional aluminium and/or copper filtration can also give a comparable dose reduction, and does not need a trebling of exposure time as with erbium.

Carbon fibre components

When first available in the late 1970s, these were plagued with mechanical stability problems. It was not uncommon to see table tops stuck together with adhesive tape where they had failed under a heavy patient. This unfortunate early history has undoubtedly led to an adverse perception of this valuable material. Modern carbon fibre is now extremely strong and can be relied upon to give many years of service.

The advantages in terms of dose reduction are not however universal. At low kV_p values such as in paediatrics, mammography and orthopaedics, the advantages are without doubt. Publications on the subject almost invariably employ a kV_p value of 60 for their comparisons. Above 65 the savings are much reduced, and above 85 they are negligible. This is due to the differences in absorption processes across the diagnostic range. At 60 kV the absorption process is predominantly photoelectric, where the extent is proportional to the cube of the atomic number of the absorber. As kV rises, Compton scatter predominates, which is proportional to density of absorber and independent of atomic number.

Carbon fibre is similar in density to plastics or aluminium but has a lower atomic number than either. On this basis carbon fibre table tops are extremely advantageous for:

- *Paediatrics* – all applications. Speedy uptake of this material should be encouraged for this work.
- *Accident and Emergency* – only where much table-top work is done; that is, equipment systems which allow ease of transfer of traumatized patients on to the X-ray table. If most trauma patients remain on a casualty trolley for their examination, a carbon fibre table top is of no benefit to them.
- *Orthopaedics and Rheumatology* – carbon fibre allows excellent contrast and improved soft tissue detail.
- *Angiography* – where kV_p is always kept low to avoid overpenetration of iodinated contrast agents.

Disadvantages

Carbon fibre table tops are extremely costly, at approximately three times the price of conventional foam sandwich types. Carbon fibre has poor shock absorption characteristics; if heavy apparatus is dropped on to such a table top, it may shatter. Repairs are also a problem. Minor damage cannot be filled in with auto repair resin (as with conventional table tops), since this would cause an artefact. Costly factory repairs are the only possibility, considerably adding to maintenance costs. The table top itself may cause an artefact in certain circumstances, where the structure of the material may be visible on radiographs.

Carbon fibre table tops offer no advantage for barium studies where kV_p is high.

Carbon fibre cassette fronts

This material approximately doubles the cost of a cassette (including screens).

Carbon fibre cassette fronts are advantageous for paediatrics, especially neonatal radiography. Savings are even greater than apparent from exposure factor reductions, due to reduced back-scatter to the baby from the cassette.

They are also advantageous for orthopaedics. Image contrast is often increased since low-energy photons may reach the film giving extra soft tissue detail.

Carbon fibre grid interspacing

This is advantageous for mammography, where grids are used with automatic exposure devices (especially in breast screening). It is also extremely useful for the rare occasions where the pregnant abdomen is X-rayed. Carbon fibre grid interspacing is very useful for any paediatric work, and in angiography where kV_p is low. However, it is of little value for barium studies, where the kilovoltage is at the higher end of the diagnostic range.

Increased focal film distances, ideally combined with non-grid technique

Here skin dose is reduced due to the inverse square law. Magnification and distortion of the image are also reduced. Exposure factors must however increase, to maintain the dose to the image receptor. When combined with air gap technique rather than a grid, dose savings are significant. Double the focus to film distance, discard the grid and use an air gap ($\approx 15\,cm$) between patient and film. This can employ the same exposure factors as the conventional technique, reducing the patient dose by as much as 70%.

Increased kilovoltage settings

This will result in reduced skin dose but, depending on the site involved, critical organ doses may increase due to additional internal scatter. Image contrast will be reduced, and this may compromise the diagnostic value of the examination. When combined with rare earth intensifying screens, where conversion efficiency may increase with kilovoltage, this technique may ultimately result in reduced patient doses.

Ultrafine collimation – slit beam techniques

Radiographic techniques which employ ultrafine collimation can offer great dose savings. The amount of scattered radiation produced is so small that a grid may be unnecessary, with additional dose savings as a result. One example is the tightly coned open mouth view of C1. Here field sizes as small as 5 × 5 cm may be used, removing the need for a grid. Slit beam techniques are a development from this. Only a tiny volume of the patient is irradiated at a time and a correspondingly tiny area of image receptor is exposed at a time, thus reducing scatter and improving image quality.

Beam-shaping filters

One can improve image quality and reduce dose by tailoring exposure for differing tissue densities in the patient. In the chest, during hilar tomography, there is a great variation in tissue density across the area of interest. The thoracic spine lies in the centre of the field, with the air-filled lungs to each side. A beam-shaping filter can even out the film density by absorbing more radiation over the lungs and less over the spine. In barium enema lateral decubitus projections, especially on more obese patients, the abdominal fat falls towards the table top, producing a very dense area near the table, with a depleted area at the top of the patient. A wedge filter can be used to great advantage to even out these differences, improving the overall image quality as well as reducing dose.

Excellent magnetic/clear lead perspex ranges are available, but these are expensive and need to be bought for each room.

This particular option offers dose reduction as well as the possibility for image enhancement, and as such should merit serious consideration.

Collimation and postcollimation

Irradiation of tissue outside the region of diagnostic interest simply adds to patient detriment without improving the results. Worse still, it can degrade the image. Image area protocols should be reviewed for common projections. Use of postcollimation (as in radiography of the lateral lumbar spine, where the region of interest and centring point lie close to the skin surface) can only serve to improve image quality as well as reduce dose.

Automatic exposure devices

(Smith et al. BIR Report 20 1989.) This equipment does not reduce radiation doses. Consistency may even be reduced compared with manual selection of factors, and skill is lost when the automatic exposure device is inappropriate or fails to function. For inexperienced operators however, consistency can be improved with this equipment.

Large field intensifiers

Use of this technology in conjunction with 100 mm photofluorographic film offers the scope for large dose reduction of up to 50% in chest radiography compared to the conventional technique. Image quality may suffer slightly, but this technology may be useful for mass screening, when any suspect case is recalled for a full-size radiograph.

Asymmetric intensifying screens

Pioneered in Sweden, using fast screens on the back and slow screens on the front (tube side) of a cassette can increase speed and improve resolution. More of the transmitted radiation is converted to produce the image, with excellent results. The slow screen enhances resolution, and the fast screen improves speed, with dose reduction as an incidental advantage (Paris, BIR Report 20 1989).

Mammography

Automatic exposure devices are vital for breast screening, where consistent results are imperative for maintaining pick-up rates, but there is room for improvement. A grid must always be used with an automatic exposure device, as it acts only as a photon counter, and cannot distinguish between scattered and image-forming photons. Consequently the dose increases by up to 40%, compared with the non-grid technique, but image quality is improved (Thilander et al. BIR Report 20 1989).

Conclusion

This has been an overview of dose-saving options. It is not intended to be complete, and as technology advances, further developments may even overshadow those listed here in terms of dose reduction impact.

This chapter does however indicate that investing heavily in dose reduction equipment does not necessarily reduce doses. Proper evaluation of the merits of these measures in a particular application is required before resources are allocated. Replacing *all* departmental cassettes and tables tops with carbon fibre will be of benefit in only a limited number of areas, and may prove costly in increased maintenance charges, as well as capital outlay.

7

Special requirements of women who are or might be pregnant

No group evokes more anxiety and concern than those women who are pregnant, those who might be pregnant and, most of all, those who turn out to have been pregnant at the time of the X-ray examination.

As many as 20% of women between the ages of 18 and 30 may be pregnant at any one time. Keeping such a statistic in mind is helpful when examining such patients.

Note: It is vital to consult the department's radiation protection adviser whenever decisions or policies regarding pregnant women are being considered. The position regarding this group is rapidly changing and it is important to ensure that the most up-to-date information is used when advising these patients. *This is of critical importance when a possible termination of pregnancy is being considered.*

Covered in this chapter is the information required in order to calculate the dose to the fetus. There is a worked example calculation of dose to the fetus, an indication of the level of dose considered to be a hazard, and which examinations are likely to impart doses at or above the threshold believed to carry an increased risk to the developing embryo.

'Are you pregnant?' posters

Every X-ray department *must* have posters on display in the waiting area requesting pregnant women to notify the staff of their pregnancy before their examination commences. Hospitals with large non-English-speaking catchment areas should also have notices translated into the various foreign languages likely

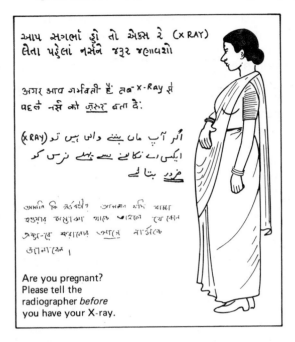

Fig. 7.1 Are you pregnant? poster.

to be encountered. Displaying the posters is not enough: we must also draw our patients' notice to them. In some countries, literacy for women is not considered to be a priority; a patient may not be able to read a notice even if it is in her own dialect. Thus the posters must be pictorial to be sure of getting the message across (Fig. 7.1).

Accidental irradiation of pregnant women

Despite the normally accepted principle that pregnancy commences on or about the 14th day post last menstrual period (LMP), it is not uncommon for women to menstruate during the first or even subsequent months of pregnancy. Additionally there are many women who menstruate on an irregular cycle. Consequently, the use of LMP and rigorous adherence to the 28-day or even the 10-day rules (see Chapter 6) may not always prevent the accidental irradiation of a fetus. Even the best-run X-ray department will occasionally, in error, carry out a radiological examination without first checking for the possibility of a coexisting pregnancy. We are all human and we all make mistakes. (It should not be forgotten that a small number of women deliberately persuade their doctors to send them for an X-ray examination to ensure that they will not experience difficulty in arranging the termination of an unwanted pregnancy.) Such incidents result in anxiety for the patient and frantic telephone calls between the general practitioner (or other clinician responsible for the patient) and the radiologist in charge of the X-ray department. The radiographer (and radiologist if it was a fluoroscopy study) who carried out the examination will experience self-recrimination until the matter is resolved.

The matter is far less unpleasant if sensible measures such as those detailed below are taken. It is not over-reacting to treat *all* female patients of childbearing age as potentially pregnant unless a good reason exists for thinking otherwise. This means practising all possible dose limitation and reduction measures for all fertile women.

Counselling the patient who is considering a termination

The International Commission on Radiological Protection (ICRP) recommended in 1984 that no patient should be advised to terminate a pregnancy due to possible radiation hazard unless the dose to the fetus was equal to or greater than 100 mGy.

In the 1988 publication *Are X-rays Safe Enough?* (Institute of Physical Science in Medicine), Dr JHE Carmichael (of the ICRP) was quoted as follows:

> International experience was that you would not consider abortion below 50 mGy and probably most people would regard 100 mGy as the appropriate figure. This does rather emphasise the need for accurate fetal dose measurements.

Radiologists are occasionally required to counsel the patient (or the referring clinician) as to the possible harm to the pregnancy and the suggested course of action. As indicated above, abortion is only considered in the highest dose procedures – barium enema, intravenous urogram, barium meal, abdominal and pelvic computed tomography scan and angiography – where an increase in the probability of malformation (over and above that naturally occurring) could have been imparted to the patient's developing fetus.

The level of dose likely to have been delivered is determined. (Chapter 4 quotes uterus doses from common X-ray examinations; see also appendix to this chapter for a worked example.)

The level at which harm could result (50–100 mGy) is quoted and compared. If the dose received was considerably lower than 50 mGy, the patient and her clinician can be reassured. If there is not a sizeable comfort margin, the method of approach must be quite different.

Where the dose is high and comparable with the levels quoted for possible consideration of a termination, the radiologist in charge of the case, along with the radiation protection adviser and the patient's clinician, will need to confer on the case. A long-wished-for pregnancy in an older woman will require different advice to that offered to a fertile, younger women who could easily embark on another pregnancy.

The probability of some kind of abnormality – be it genetic (before pregnancy) or congenital (during pregnancy) – is already high in the general population, at about 1 in 200 live births. Depending on the timing of the radiation dose in the pregnancy (which can be ascertained using ultrasound facilities) the risks can be categorized as follows.

Dose received during the first 4 weeks post LMP

The dose received during the first 4 weeks post LMP will either terminate the pregnancy, or the fetus may recover completely. Continuation as a viable pregnancy suggests that the fetus has come through unscathed. Some cells were killed, but the common pool of pluripotential cells has replaced those destroyed, and the development continues normally. Organs have not yet started to differentiate. The conceptus is not more radiosensitive than an unfertilized ovum.

Dose received 8–15 weeks post LMP

At 8–16 weeks post LMP, while organogenesis (individual organ formation) is in progress, the radiation dose may result in various types of organ damage. The exact nature will depend upon the particular organ being formed at the precise moment of irradiation. For example, between 8 and 15 weeks is the critical stage for causation of severe mental retardation since the forebrain is forming at that time.

At 100 mGy, no detectable decrease in IQ is seen over the general distribution, but when larger doses are received *in utero*, an increase in the numbers of seriously mentally retarded children is seen. At this stage, if a fetus is irradiated to a high dose, a decrease of approximately 30 IQ points per 100 mGy may be expected. The risk is 1 in 2500 per mGy above a threshold of 250 mGy.

Dose received 15 weeks or more post LMP

From 15 weeks postconception the most likely form of damage is mental retardation, with an IQ reduction of 30 IQ points per gray (see also Chapter 2). The ICRP recommendations of 1990 advise that there is no significant risk of mental retardation outside the period 8–25 weeks.

As far as cancer risk is concerned, the excess is about 1 in 5000 per mGy (from the results of the Oxford survey). The risk for the first 3 months is about three times that for the last 3 months of pregnancy, because the early embryo is most radiosensitive at that time.

Dose received at 32 weeks or later post LMP

Beyond 32 weeks, the pregnancy is clearly visible and hopefully the uterus will be well-protected. At this stage the major concern is increased cancer risk to the child during childhood or early adult life.

Cancer risk due to irradiation at any stage in pregnancy

There are approximately 50 cases of childhood cancer per 100 000 live births in the population generally. This compares with 75 childhood cancers per 100 000 children who were irradiated during pregnancy. As a consequence the ARSAC secretariat recommends radiation doses of no more than 0.5 mGy be allowed to the fetus unless there are extremely good clinical reasons.

Counselling the patient where the dose is lower than the risk threshold

When counselling such a patient, it is as well to point out that even though the coexisting pregnancy was unknown, in your department *all* patients are X-rayed with the utmost care and attention to dose-limiting methods. If – and hopefully this is always the case – cone marks are visible on the film, and where the uterus lies outside the radiation field, it can be most helpful to show the films to the patient in order to demonstrate that no X-rays actually reached the baby. Additionally, the dissimilarities between X-rays and nuclear weapons, atomic fallout or nuclear power station releases should be stressed. When appropriate, the patient may be reassured by comments such as 'X-rays cause very little change in the body – they mostly pass straight through you, that is why they reach the film', or 'The radioactive fallout from nuclear weapons stays in the body for months or years, unlike the radiation from our X-ray machines, which is very much like light, and is gone when I take my finger off the button'.

Case study

A distressed patient arrived at the X-ray department one morning. She asked to see the radiographer in charge. The lady then proceeded to tell the superintendent that 10 days earlier she had injured her shoulder and been sent for an X-ray examination. She had now found out she was pregnant and was extremely anxious about any possible injury to her baby.

The films were traced and brought to the reception area. They were then shown to the patient. Crisp cone marks (a round extension cone had been used) were visible on the films with no penumbra around them. The patient was reassured that radiation

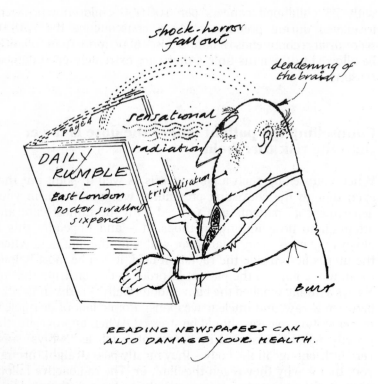

READING NEWSPAPERS CAN ALSO DAMAGE YOUR HEALTH.

had reached only her shoulder and not her baby, and went home confident that the baby had not been injured.

Conclusion

When dealing with such incidents bear in mind the following points. Pregnant women can become extremely emotional and anxious due to hormonal changes, and should be treated with compassion and patience. Pregnancy is a worrying time, involving numerous visits to the hospital, which one normally associates with illness. It is therefore not surprising that our patients constantly imagine something is wrong.

The horror stories in the press about damaged babies and radiation dangers have in some cases been vastly exaggerated, but have resulted in serious fears in our patients. These fears must be treated with respect and time should be taken to help the patient understand the true situation.

Never dismiss a patient's question with a flippant response. She may go over and over your words in her mind, as she becomes progresively more anxious. Apart from insulting her intelligence, there is the possibility of a regrettable response all over the local papers within days, damaging the reputation of the hospital and the radiographic profession at large.

Remember that ionizing radiation can be considerably less damaging to the fetus than smoking (even passive smoking), many types of chemicals, drugs (whether legal or illegal) and poor maternal nutrition (lack of vitamin B is widely believed to be a factor in some neural tube defects). (NCRP 96, 1989 *Comparative Carcinogenicity of Ionizing Radiation and Chemicals*.)

X-ray of the patient who is known to be pregnant

Professionalism is vital here. In order to trust the radiographer's skill the patient needs to see someone in whom she can have confidence.

Outline to the patient all the measures being taken to limit the dose to her baby. Use an oversize cassette if the fetus lies outside the field, and endeavour to get clear collimation visible on each film and show this to the patient afterwards to reassure her. Use appropriate gonad protection and explain each dose limitation or reduction step followed. Use beam-limiting cones if appropriate to reduce any irradiation of areas outside the region of interest.

Chest radiography

Explain that the lungs are full of air and that the X-rays pass straight through, thus very little dose is required to produce the film, and virtually nothing gets to the baby. Try to avoid using a high kilovoltage technique in the examination of the pregnant patient's chest; increased internal scatter is generated, more extrafocal radiation is produced and both further irradiate the fetus. Obligatory use of a grid with high kV_p further increases the dose.

Table 7.1 MEAN FETAL DOSE ADMINISTERED BY VARIOUS X-RAY TECH-NIQUES

Technique	Mean fetal dose (mGy)
Lateral pelvimetry	
Standard screens, crossed-hatch grid	5.800
Rare earth screens, smaller field size, single grid	0.079
Faster rare earth screens	0.066
Air gap rather than grid	0.016
Carbon fibre cassette, grid and table top	0.014
Anteroposterior orthodiagraphic for interspinous measurement (rare now)	
Standard-speed screens	2.400
Rare earth screens, no grid, smaller field size	0.031
Faster rare earth screens	0.015
Carbon fibre cassette, grid interspace, table top	0.012

(ref: Are X-Rays Safe Enough I.P.S.M. 1988)

Pelvimetry

Where a computed tomography (CT) scanner is available, scanography is the examination of choice; otherwise the fetal dose in lateral pelvimetry can be markedly reduced by various measures. Tight collimation, rare earth intensifying screens, air gap technique and carbon fibre components are all helpful (Table 7.1). The advantages of carbon fibre are lost however if high kV_p technique is used: $55{-}60\,kV_p$ should be considered a maximum for this work.

The remarkably reduced doses seen in Table 7.1 are a reflection of improved techniques and advances in technology. The dose reductions do however rely heavily upon total accuracy in technique, proper shielding of the fetus and do not include repeats. In the real world, this is not always possible.

Low-dose pelvimetry using a CT scanner

Digital radiography using a CT scanner for pelvimetry offers a real alternative to standard radiographic techniques. It is more pleasant for the patient, faster to perform, and eliminates the need for repeat exposures. CT pelvimetry offers dose reductions for the whole examination of up to 90% compared with standard techniques. The whole examination gives a mean fetal dose of 0.010 mGy (n.b. quoted figure has been extrapolated to make it comparable with those from other references. Original paper quoted ovary, not uterus dose.) (Lotz et al., 1987.)

A single CT slice through the pelvis for interspinous measurement gives approximately 5 mGy to the fetus.

The patient who might be pregnant

Whenever a patient insists that she is *not* pregnant, have her sign to confirm this on the X-ray request form. This will be valuable evidence in the defence of a radiographer or radiologist accused of failing to ask the patient if she is pregnant. Such accusations are made from time to time and the whole experience is thoroughly unpleasant for anyone involved. The positive act of signing a document tends to make patients think more carefully about their answer to the pregnancy question, and may help ensure that the true facts are known to the staff. If the patient thinks that she might be pregnant, check that the referring clinician is aware of this.

Are the symptoms in fact due to an undiagnosed pregnancy? Nausea, change in bowel habit and lower abdominal pain can all be associated with early pregnancy.

Could the examination wait until later in the pregnancy when organogenesis is complete?

Could a pregnancy test be performed to confirm whether or not she is pregnant? If the examination must continue, it is important to involve a radiologist. The examination could be modified to take account of the patient's condition and limited numbers of films may be indicated. Alternatively it may be possible to use ultrasound instead or other non-ionizing radiation procedures. (eg IVU replaced by U/S – BJR Feb. 1991. Ultrasound of the breast replacing mammography etc.).

Appendix

Worked example of dose to the fetus

Note: In this appendix the obsolete unit the röntgen (R) has been used for exposure, because:

1. The röntgen is the unit indicated on the front of many radiation output units, and is the unit used in many departmental quality assurance radiation output measurements. Comparison of these values can thus be made to the tube outputs in readers' own departments without the need for calculations.
2. The use of röntgen for these calculations makes the required concepts easier to understand.
3. The worked example is taken from a classic document where the röntgen is used, and converting the data to SI units is not acceptable to the author (NCRP 54, 1977).

Reproduced by kind permission of the National Council for Radiological Protection and Measurements, Bethesda, Maryland, USA.

Table 7A.1 FETAL DOSES PER RÖNTGEN FOR COMMON EXAMINATIONS

Examination	Mean fetal dose (mGy per R exposure)
AP pelvis	2.83 (also venogram)
Pelvis lateral	0.39
AP hip (one side)	2.00
Femur one side AP	0.48 (also venogram)
Abdomen AP*	2.65
Abdomen PA	1.30
Lumbar spine AP	2.50
Lumbar spine lateral	0.27
Lumbar spine lateral L5–S1	0.39
Thoracic spine AP	0.008
Thoracic spine lateral	0.002
Full spine (chiropractic) AP	3.08 (C, T and L spine)
Chest PA	0.012
Chest AP	0.013
Chest lateral	0.005
(Skull, cervical spine, shoulder, humerus)	< 0.0001

AP = Anteroposterior; PA = posteroanterior
*Abdomen includes intravenous urogram, barium enema and angiography.
Note: assuming total filtration of 2.5 mm of aluminium in the beam. All data are quoted for exposure at 1 m focus detector distance.
For *three phase X-ray equipment* the exposures are approximately: $80 \, kV_p = 6.5 \, mR/mAs$ at 1 m ($60 \, kV_p = 4.0/70 = 5.3/90 = 9.0$)
For *single-phase equipment*, the figure is lower at: $80 \, kV_p = 4.4 \, mR/mAs$ at 1 m ($60 = 1.9/70 = 3.2/90 = 6.4$)

Example calculation

An average-sized woman undergoes four anteroposterior (AP) radiographs of the pelvis in early pregnancy.

The patient's anteroposterior thickness is 26 cm.

The focus to film distance is 1 m.

The tube potential is $80\,kV_p$.

Equipment used is a three-phase generator.

Total filtration on the X-ray tube is 2.5 mm aluminium.

Tube current setting is 300 mA.

Exposure time for each radiograph is 0.2 s.

To overestimate the final dose slightly, and to make the mathematics simpler to follow, the figure of 10 mR/mAs has been used.

$300\,mA \times 0.2\,s \times 4\,views \times 10\,mR/mAs = 2.4\,R$.

In this case, there is a 5-cm gap between film and patient, allowing for the bucky and mattress. The source to skin distance thus becomes:

AP patient thickness = 26 cm.

Film to back of patient = 5 cm.

Film to front of patient is = 26 + 5 = 31 cm.

Source to front of patient is = 100 cm − 31 cm = 69 cm

Exposure in air at 100 cm = 2.4 R.

Exposure in air at 69 cm = $[\dfrac{(100)^2}{(69)} \times 2.4\,R] = 5.04\,R$.

From Table 7A.1 the dose to the uterus (fetus in early pregnancy) for an AP pelvis for an average patient is $\simeq 2.83\,mGy/R$.

For this example the figures give: $5.04\,R \times 2.83\,mGy/R = 14.26\,mGy$ in total.

This is well below the 50–100 mGy threshold quoted earlier in this chapter.

Conclusion for the worked example

One would not recommend a termination of pregnancy for the patient in the case quoted above. Reference to Table 4.4 shows the mean uterus dose from an AP pelvis X-ray to be 1.55 mGy. For four such exposures, the total would be 6.2 mGy. The mean doses given in Table 4.4 all assume optimum technique; maximum figures in the same table are 4.5 times higher. The result shown here is commensurate with the sort of conditions encountered in real incidents, and gives a value which is likely to be encountered in investigations of pregnant patients.

Note: This worked example has been somewhat simplified to make it easy to follow. It is strongly recommended that any reader seriously involved in counselling pregnant patients consult the radiation protection adviser for detailed guidance. The proper handling of such an incident may well involve recreating the original examination and making careful measurements. Such incidents may ultimately be the subject of legal action, and reading this book does not necessarily confer competence in this field.

Suppose there is a 5% increase in possible abnormality due to a radiation dose. If every fetus so irradiated were terminated, for every 100 irradiated pregnancies 95 normal babies would be destroyed to prevent the birth of five possibly abnormal ones. Approximately one in every 200 live births has a serious abnormality without any added risk factors.

Conclusion

As a general rule of thumb, the 50–100 mGy fetal dose will only be encountered in studies involving several views of the pelvis or abdomen, i.e. barium enema, intravenous urogram, abdominal angiography, abdominal or pelvic CT and skeletal surveys, where even with low-dose techniques one might approach or exceed the threshold figures quoted. That said, where poor technique (no rare earth screens, repeats, short focus to film distance) is used, fetal doses for even the lower-dose examinations will be high – up to 40 times those achievable with good technique.

Average skin doses for common examinations should be measured in every X-ray room in the department and made available to the staff. This will help ensure that doses given are *ALARP* (as low as reasonably practicable).

8

Paediatric radiation protection

The radiographic examination of children and babies differs from that of adults in several important ways. Even the most experienced radiographer may find paediatric work daunting. Ideally all children would be sent to a specialist paediatric hospital. Sadly this is not always possible. Efforts must be made to ensure that the standards of paediatric radiography are optimized.

Training

For the radiographer

The most important and effective measure that can be taken to improve the diagnostic and safety standards in paediatric radiography is training. This must not be seen as a small part of the basic training, but as an extremely important ongoing aid to safety and good practice in general.

A paediatric radiography specialist radiographer should be appointed in every X-ray department where children are examined. This person attends study days, keeps up to date with relevant journal articles and provides regular teach-in sessions on paediatric radiography for colleagues. A certificate of competence in paediatric radiography should be developed, as has been introduced in mammography.

For the radiologist

The specialist nature of paediatric radiology demands very special skills from the reporting radiologist, and ongoing training should be provided. The nuances of epiphyseal bone development in children, with the variations in different ethnic groups, often demand extraordinary skill to avoid the need for comparison

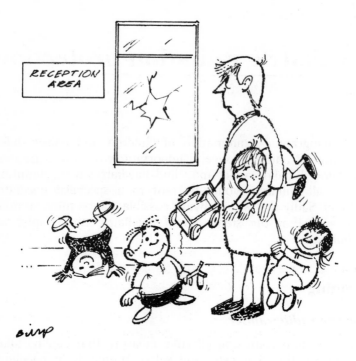

views of the opposite side in, for example, wrist injuries in small children, doubling the dose to the patient.

Indications

The pathologies for which babies and children are referred are often quite different from those affecting adults. In many cases it is impossible to locate the precise site of the trouble due to immaturity or inability to communicate. Only a proper knowledge of the pathologies affecting small children and their radiographic or radiological significance can ensure that the correct examination is performed in each case.

There are a number of excellent volumes on this subject, such as Catherine Gyll's *Paediatric Diagnostic Imaging* and at least one copy should reside on the shelf next to the departmental '*Kitty Clark*'.

Non-accidental injury

The tragic epidemic of violence against children has resulted in large numbers of requests for skeletal surveys for non-accidental injury. Such requests demand special skills from an experienced radiographer in terms of discretion when dealing with the parents, sensitivity when dealing with the child, and absolute accuracy, with attention to detail, when producing the radiographs. Failure to mark the films with correct right or left markers, name or date can render the radiographs inadmissible in court, and as such completely fail to satisfy the purpose of the examination. Such films have to be repeated, doubling the dose to the patient, even if the first attempt was technically adequate.

Radionuclide imaging is another modality for the investigation of non-accidental injury in small children. Providing that the child's bladder is emptied frequently (see Chapter 12), the dose for a bone scan is similar to that for a skeletal survey, and there is no extra radiation dose if a view has to be repeated. An additional benefit of radionuclide imaging is that bruising (a frequent feature in non-accidental injury) is also apparent on the images, and can be a useful diagnostic feature.

The 'babygram'

The practice of radiographing a whole child on one cassette may appear to reduce the dose to the child, simply because fewer exposures are made. The radiation dose to the child may be up to 40% greater for the 'babygram' compared to a series of tightly collimated separate views of each limb or part examined.

Parents

The parents can be of enormous help to the radiographer, both in comforting the child and in helping to immobilize him or her for the examination. Where a parent is involved in this way, the radiation protection of that person is extremely important. Always check that the mother is not pregnant. If she is, do not allow her to hold the child for the radiographic exposure, but do encourage her to remain in the room, safely behind the lead glass window of a protective screen.

It is vital to reassure her of the negligible dose rates in this position, even if she expresses no interest, since she may become worried later and suffer anxiety until she has been able to speak to a member of the X-ray staff.

It is helpful if the child is able to see the mother at all times. If she holds the infant facing her whilst donning her lead rubber apron anxiety can be considerably reduced. (Gyll, Handbook of Paediatric Radiography.)

During chest radiography, to ensure that the film is not rotated, the supporting adult needs to stand directly behind the child, holding the arms truly vertical. In this case, partially attenuated primary radiation could come through the cassette and strike the helper. A 0.5-mm lead rubber apron (or two 0.25-mm aprons worn together) should be provided. Tight collimation and use of a correctly sized gonad shield are also extremely important for such an examination.

An image of the supporting adult's hands should never appear on a radiograph of a child. Protective gloves and tight collimation should always be used to avoid this. Not only is unnecessary irradiation bad practice, but the presence of the parental phalanges may distract the radiologist when the films are reported.

Protection of the child

Because of the radiosensitivity of small children, and the child-bearing capacity of all youngsters, radiation protection for the young patient takes on great importance. There is increased opportunity for expression of delayed radiogenic cancers in the young. Also their smaller size brings all organs closer to or within the useful beam, giving a higher overall exposure per radiograph than for adults. (ref: *Patient Dosimetry Techniques in Diagnostic Radiology*. IPSM Report 53, 1988.)

X-ray departments devoted exclusively to the examination of children are quite different in design to those used for adults. In the general department, the vast majority of patients are elderly, the critical group for protection are the staff, and undercouch screening is usually the system of choice. Overcouch fluoroscopy units, with their lower skin dose to the patient, are of considerable benefit in paediatric radiology. Such equipment does however result in far higher staff doses, and is usually only installed as a remote-control facility. Remote-control radiographic equipment is not appropriate for small children who need the reassuring presence of an adult during their examination. Fluoroscopy examinations on children should be performed without a grid in most cases, and the details of the technique altered to suit the patient's age and pathology.

Immobilization

Equipment is available to restrain the child and immobilize him or her for the examination. These accessories include cradles, bucky bands, Velcro straps, beanbags and headrests. Total restraint is really a last resort, but may be necessary for cases where speed is critical. Use of restraining equipment can induce a terrible fear of the X-ray department, causing serious problems if the child ever returns for repeat examinations.

Where all else fails, general anaesthesia is the only practical option for immobilization, especially for computed tomography, angiography and magnetic resonance imaging. (General anaesthesia is used extensively in veterinary radiography where immobilization presents similar difficulties.)

Teddies

Assisting a toddler to radiograph a teddy is useful in reassuring the patient, and may result in a superior film first time. Although there is no genetically significant dose, gonad protection should be used.

Breast protection

The breasts of female children and particularly adolescents (due to intense glandular development) are extremely radiosensitive and should receive similar consideration during radiography as the gonads. Great care should be taken totally to exclude the breast from the irradiated field in examinations such as the shoulder, humerus and abdominal studies, including intravenous urography. A sheet of lead rubber strategically placed will considerably reduce dose to the immature breast. The appearance of an unintended mammogram on a radiograph of the humerus is not uncommon (Gyll, 1990, personal communication) and should be avoided at all costs.

Gonad protection

Gonad protection should be employed for all children undergoing X-ray examination, except where it may obscure diagnostic information. Possibility of misplacement is simply not a reason to leave it off. There are occasions where gonad protection may be inappropriate, such as the *first* visit for evaluation of congenital dysplasia of the hip, on *female* children. Such cases should be carefully considered and guidelines prepared. It may be useful to tape gonad shields in place when examining small children. When examinations of the extremities, skull, shoulder or knee joints are undertaken, gonad protection should always be used. The few extra moments taken will not appreciably lengthen the examination time, and the attending parent will be reassured. When the older child or adolescent is examined, an explanation of the purpose of the protective equipment is of tremendous interest and may well distract him or her from the discomfort of the examination.

Male children

Ask the patient to pull his pants down over the symphysis pubis, but still covering the testes and penis. This allows the testes to fall away from the pubic bone, but still keeps them warm. The pants can then help support the gonad shield across the thighs.

A premature baby may have undescended testes; give lower abdomen protection as for a girl. Note also that it is not necessary to see the lower pelvis on a film to indicate the position of an umbilical artery catheter.

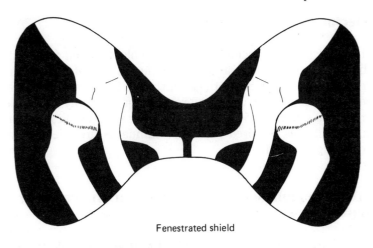

Fenestrated shield

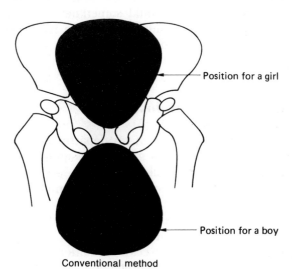

Position for a girl

Position for a boy

Conventional method

Fig. 8.1 Methods of gonad shielding.

Female children

The ovaries can be virtually anywhere within the pelvic cavity (NCRP 68, 1981), but use of a pelvic-cavity gonad shield, cut to size from a radiograph so that it covers the sacrum (Gyll, 1987), reduces internal scatter within the area, and thus dose to the ovaries, wherever they may be (Fig. 8.1).

Special techniques

There are several special techniques available to aid diagnosis in children and babies. Examples include the use of a carbonated drink to fill the stomach with gas during an intravenous urogram; angled renal window view; anteroposterior view only for shoulder injury; no separate L5–S1 film for lumbar spine studies. Continuous training is required to ensure standards are adequate and knowledge current.

Atlas of epiphyseal development for the casualty department

The need for comparison views of the uninjured side in orthopaedic injuries in children could sometimes be avoided if an appropriate text is made available to the casualty department. This is a clinical issue outside the scope of this text, but worthy of consideration.

Genetically significant dose

Unlike much of the work in the X-ray department, all the studies performed on children carry a genetically significant dose. This means that all children could potentially go on to produce children themselves and as such their dose must be considered as possibly affecting future generations. This is in contrast to examinations on elderly adults or adults of childbearing capacity who have completed their families.

Therefore all available resources for radiation protection should be directed towards paediatric protection as a priority. Carbon fibre cassette fronts should be used for paediatric examinations and all the other dose reduction measures listed in Chapter 6 should be made available for these patients. One should however keep in mind the different methods used in the examination of children compared to adults, when purchasing protection equipment. One particular example is the fact that small children are rarely examined using a secondary radiation grid, due to the fact that their body parts are small; far less scattered radiation is generated than would be the case with an adult. Carbon fibre grid interspacing material, and possibly even table tops, are therefore of less value for dose reduction for these patients and should not figure as the top priority.

Artefacts

The lower kilovoltages used in paediatric radiography may result in greater problems with artefacts. Fireproofing treatment of nightclothes may show up on the radiograph; embroidery and other decorations may be visible from underwear. It is wise to examine carefully any clothing worn during the examination, or better still to remove the patient's garments and radiograph the child in a radiolucent X-ray gown. The laundry may need to be instructed not to use starch on paediatric X-ray gowns, because the low kilovoltages may make starch artefacts more likely.

Special care baby unit (SCBU) radiography

Premature babies undergoing intensive therapy often require repeated radiographs, especially when in respiratory distress due to lung immaturity. Doses given in such cases should be minimized as far as possible. Quality assurance on the mobile unit used for this work should take place more frequently than on other mobiles in the hospital. Carbon fibre cassette fronts and superfast intensifying screens should be employed. High-output generators with reliable timers are indicated. Gonad and thyroid shields can be used on top of the incubator to protect the tiny patient.

The assistance of a member of the nursing staff to immobilize and support the tiny patient may well be necessary.

Staff doses

Doses to SCBU staff assisting with premature baby radiography are negligible, due to the low kilovoltages and small field sizes employed. The skin dose to the trunk (without a lead rubber apron) is approximately $3\,\mu Gy$ per examination. With a lead rubber apron the dose drops to $1\,\mu Gy$ per examination. The exposure to the eyes is approximately 5 μGy, and that to the hands is about 10 μGy. A member of the SCBU staff could assist with such examinations (wearing a lead rubber protective apron) up to 5000 times per year, before reaching the dose limit for the general public. This duty is non-hazardous.

To satisfy the ALARA principle, however, the work should be shared out between as many non-pregnant staff (and parents) as possible, and records kept of such duties to ensure an even spread.

Conclusion

The considerably greater radiosensitivities of the organs and bone marrow in children indicates that we should redouble our efforts in the radiation protection area for this group.

9

Advice on radiation protection and action in overexposure cases

Radiographers and radiologists should be encouraged to seek advice and information on radiation protection at all times. Staff are then well prepared to answer the questions posed by patients and fellow hospital professionals. They are also in a better position to respond to emergency situations.

Advice on overexposure

Accidents involving ionizing radiation occur from time to time. It is advisable to know in advance where to get the necessary advice, so that it is to hand when an incident arises. Such emergencies invariably take place at 4.55 on the Friday before a bank holiday, when the radiation protection adviser (RPA) is on a lecture tour of subsaharan Africa.

The first person to approach for advice on any aspect of radiation protection in the X-ray department is the radiation protection supervisor (RPS). This is usually the superintendent radiographer, but may be another senior member of staff. The RPS is responsible for day-to-day issues involving radiation safety, and he or she will be able to deal with most minor problems. When this person is unavailable, and the issue is urgent, it is not inappropriate to approach the RPA directly.

The identity and contact numbers for the RPA can usually be found:

1. In the local rules for the X-ray department.
2. Displayed on the nuclear medicine department notice board.
3. In the minutes of the radiological protection committee meetings.

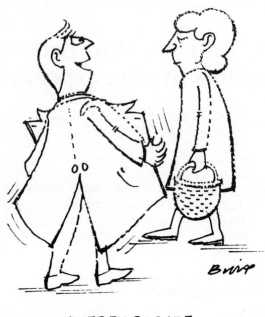

... OVEREXPOSURE ....

4. From the switchboard of your hospital as part of the emergency contingency plans for a radiation incident.

Consultant radiologists, particularly those who hold an Administration of Radioactive Substances Advisory Committee (ARSAC) licence have great in depth knowledge of radiation safety, and are in a position to offer expert guidance. Many have also been involved in running training courses for other clinicians, such as those required under the UK Ionizing Radiation Regulations' 1988 core of knowledge. The radiological profession generally has taken a leading role in ensuring other medical specialties improve their knowledge of radiation safety.

Other sources of guidance are: other X-ray departments, the physics department at a neighbouring or associated hospital, and the local radiography training school. The following organizations are able to offer guidance in different areas of the field: National Radiological Protection Board (or equivalent in other countries); UK Atomic Energy Authority (or equivalent);

and European Community Radiation and Radiation Protection Division.

Availability of publications

Information is readily available from the many publications in the field of radiation protection. Every X-ray department should offer its staff a basic library of reference books on the subject, for interest as well as satisfying legal obligations to patients and other staff. These books are helpful to radiographers studying for post-diploma qualifications, as well as radiologists working towards their Fellowship of the Royal College of Radiologists Part One examinations.

Suggested texts are listed in the Bibliography and Further Reading.

Deputy RPS

It is advisable that at least one member of the staff, in addition to the RPS, develops a special interest in radiation protection, attending courses and reading relevant papers in the journals (such as *British Journal of Radiology* and *Radiography Today* in the UK). This person can then deputize when the RPS is away.

The RPS is often the superintendent radiographer, under heavy pressure with a wide range of responsibilities. Whilst not a legal obligation, it can be extremely helpful to arrange a deputy; this can aid the department as well as the career progress of the individual.

We have a duty to our patients to make a commitment to radiation protection, and X-ray department management should encourage this.

How to deal with overexposure

The word overexposure conjures up images of the American television series where a research scientist overdoses himself

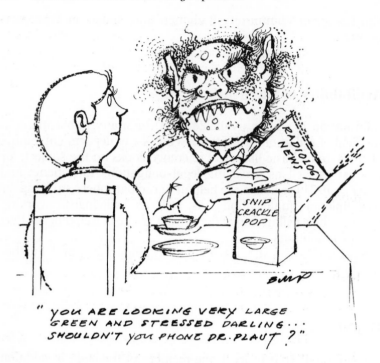

"YOU ARE LOOKING VERY LARGE GREEN AND STRESSED DARLING... SHOULDN'T YOU PHONE DR. PLAUT?"

with gamma radiation and then becomes large and green whenever stressed. Such an outcome is not possible from any overdose involving diagnostic X-ray equipment (or anything else).

What is an overexposure?

Strictly speaking, this is any radiation exposure which is found to have been much greater than originally intended, due to equipment malfunction or misuse. Such an event is extremely unlikely but does occur in various circumstances. The following provides some examples of genuine cases; it is not intended to be exhaustive.

1. The X-ray unit exposure fails to terminate and this is not noticed for several minutes. (Always check the mA meter to ensure exposure has terminated. The X-ray tube could overheat and implode, with possible danger.)

2. The screening foot pedal on the fluoroscopy unit becomes caught under a trolley wheel or under the table itself when vertical. Screening continues unnoticed for several minutes while staff prepare for the next case. (Always move the screening pedal to a safe position after each case. If necessary, replace the foot pedal with the hooded type.)
3. Two X-ray tubes are operated from the same generator and control panel. The wrong tube is selected, consequently the wrong patient as well as a radiographer are irradiated. (If necessary, initiate a policy of deselecting both tubes after every exposure, so that the operator must positively select a tube before exposing. Alternatively it is possible to fit a second exposure button to the panel.)
4. The mobile C-arm image intensifier is set up for use in the operating theatre. It is later discovered that the screening pedal had been caught under cable in its holder, and had been screening for several minutes. (Ensure the unit is never switched on until the radiographer arrives to start the case. Screening pedals are to be packed away carefully with the cable.)
5. A second exposure is initiated on the dental X-ray unit if the finger is not removed from the hand switch immediately after exposure is complete. (Watch the 'X-rays on' light.)

Action to take for overexposure involving a fluoroscopy unit

Immediately make notes of all available details of the incident. Note approximate field size, if the unit was on automatic kV_p and mA setting, or manually selected factors (if the latter, it may be necessary to reconstruct the case using phantoms to ascertain the likely exposure factors). Note the distance of any personnel from the unit, and the position of the patient (if any) in the beam. Make notes of the identity of the personnel and patient where appropriate. Note the build of the patient. Were any of the staff (or patient) in the room pregnant or possibly pregnant? Any monitored personnel should have their dosimeters sent off immediately for evaluation and the results must be included in the report.

Draft a report of the incident and send one copy to the RPS, one copy to the RPA and keep one copy for reference. If a radiologist was present, the recorded technical details will need to be made available for the radiological report.

If the incident was due to an equipment malfunction, rather than user error, the unit must not be used until repaired. It may also be necessary to report the fault to the Health and Safety Executive (HSE) and possibly also to the Department of Health (or equivalent in other countries). If it is due to a design error, it may be the subject of a hazard warning notice sent to all users.

Action to take for a general radiographic unit

Note field size, focus to film distance, table top to film distance, thickness of mattress and the patient's build (to determine the focus to skin surface distance). Note the exposure factors set and the approximate duration of exposure time. Were any repeat radiographs taken? Note the position of the patient, his or her age, identity and referring clinician or practitioner.

A copy of the films may be needed by the RPA to assist in determining the exposure received by the patient. Immediately after the incident is the best time to record the details, when they are fresh in everyone's minds. A detailed diagram of the room can be very helpful to the RPA in such cases.

There is currently no firm recommendation as to what radiation dose should be given to a patient for a particular examination. The mean dose figures quoted in NRPB R200 are a useful guide, but do not cover all procedures.

The actual doses received, particularly in fluoroscopic and angiographic procedures, are highly variable and need expert physics guidance to assess accurately.

If an exposure is much greater than intended due to an equipment or other technical fault, and exceeds the intended exposure by more than the factors specified by the HSE (Table 9.1), then the incident *must* be reported to the HSE (this is a legal requirement). The RPA will determine the actual dose received, and then decide whether or not the incident requires reporting. For the purposes of notification, the guidelines are applied as appropriate to: dose; mA; activity administered; dose area product; time; and volume of tissue irradiated or whatever measure is available and broadly representative of patient exposure. Professional judgement (by the RPA) is essential in determining the effect on patient exposure for diagnostic X-ray

Table 9.1 CRITERIA FOR NOTIFICATION OF CERTAIN INCIDENTS INVOLV-
ING MEDICAL EXPOSURE

Type of examination or treatment	*Guideline multiplying factor*
Extremities, skull, chest, dentals, elbow, knee, shoulder and other simple examinations Nuclear medicine examinations where intended $H_E < 0.5$ mSv e.g. ^{51}Cr (EDTA) GFR – glomerular filtration rate measurements	20
Mammography, abdomen, lumbar spine, pelvis and all other examinations not indicated in this table Nuclear medicine studies where intended $H_E < 5$ mSv > 0.5 mSv e.g. ^{99m}Tc MAA – macro-aggregates or microspheres lung imaging.	10
Barium enema, meal, intravenous urogram, angiography and other fluoroscopy procedures Digital radiology and computed tomography Nuclear medicine where intended $H_E > 5$ mSv e.g. ^{201}Tl (myocardial imaging)	3
Radionuclide therapy e.g. ^{131}I (any administration)	1.2

H_E = Effective dose equivalent; EDTA = ethylenediaminetetraacetic acid
(Reproduced by kind permission of the Controller of Her Majesty's Stationery
Office)

equipment which does not give a postexposure read-out of tube-
loading factors and does not allow the exposure factors to be
selected. The factors are given in terms of the ratio of *suspected*
(or actual) exposure over *intended* exposure. The figures quoted
are those published by the HSE in 1992, superseding earlier draft
criteria.

Purpose of reporting overexposure incidents

Such reporting enables the HSE to monitor hazards on a national
basis and act to reduce risks by recommending a nationwide
review of policy, practice and equipment.

As can be seen from a brief perusal of the multiplying factors,
one or two repeated films will not take the levels to that
approaching the figures quoted. The measures do *not* apply
to cases where films are repeated due to *operator* error or
misjudgement. It is hoped that personnel who frequently repeat

particular examinations due to error would endeavour to seek training to remedy this particular area of weakness.

Action in cases involving a pregnant woman

Detailed guidance is given in Chapter 7.

Useful information

In an emergency you may need to contact the RPA and RPS. RPA for this department is tel ....
RPS for this department is tel ....
   You may need to refer to the local rules, and produce evidence of when you last read this document (a legal obligation). Whereabouts of local rules ....
I read and understood the local rules on ....
....
....
....

See also Chapter 10.

10
Statutory responsibilities

In the UK, work with ionizing radiation is governed by several pieces of legislation:

- Health and Safety at Work Act 1974
- The Ionizing Radiation Regulations 1985
- The European Communities Act 1972 led to the publication of the Ionizing Radiation Regulations 1988 (Protection of Persons undergoing Medical Examination and Treatment or POPUMET or IRR 88).

The aim of IRR 88 was to keep doses as low as reasonably practicable whilst maintaining the clinical value of the X-ray examination.

IRR 85 covers all users of ionizing radiation, including manufacture of nuclear weapons and fuel reprocessing (involving terabecquerel quantities) as well as users of a few kilobecquerels in a hospital laboratory. The regulations are thus necessarily legalistic and sometimes inappropriate to the hospital environment. Further documents have appeared to help clarify and apply the law to the practical situation. The *Approved Code of Practice* (which has a legal standing) is a more accessible document with practical applications. The third in the series, however, the *Guidance Notes* (prepared by the National Radiological Protection Board, Health and Safety Executive (HSE) and Departments of Health of England, Scotland, Wales and Northern Ireland) is an extremely useful 'how-to' handbook which serves as a reference manual on good safety practice.

Use of radioactive materials

In all countries the use of radioactive materials is closely controlled by legislation, and governmental inspectorates. In the

UK, radioactive materials usage is governed by the Radioactive Substances Act 1960. The Department of the Environment (DoE) operates a system of pollution inspectors who must be satisfied about good practice and facilities before they will issue authorizations to store, use and dispose of radioactive materials. Before commencing operations, the intending user must complete a form RSA 1 to register the holding of radioactive materials. (Crown immunity enabled most National Health Service hospitals to avoid this part of the requirements; however, many have now lost this exemption in taking trust status.) If the user intends to dispose of any radioactive materials, a form RSA 3 is required. The application form is lengthy and requires considerable effort to complete. The information required includes the following:

- National grid map reference of the hospital.
- Make and age of incinerators; whether they have after-burners.
- Location of hospital sewerage supply outflow. Is it into a river or the sea? National grid map reference of outflow point.

Proper completion requires several weeks' work and since 1 April 1991, a fee from the pollution inspectorate for it to be read. Submission of such a form – be it a new application or a revision to an existing authorization (also chargeable) – usually results in a visit from the pollution inspectorate.

If the radioactive materials are to be administered to patients, the consultant clinician under whose clinical direction the work takes place will need to apply for an Administration of Radioactive Substances Advisory Committee (ARSAC) licence. Before such a licence is granted, the applicant needs to complete a lengthy form, countersigned by the radiation protection adviser (RPA), demonstrating sufficient knowledge and experience in radiation protection and the intended clinical procedure. The requirements are most easily satisfied if the clinician has attended a certified 'core of knowledge' radiation protection course. These courses are held regularly at various centres throughout the UK. The situation is similar in other European Community countries.

Once furnished with the ARSAC licence, the holder can delegate the work to named competent individuals who also hold a 'core of knowledge' or IRR 88 certificate. Such delegation requires an authorization letter from the ARSAC licence holder

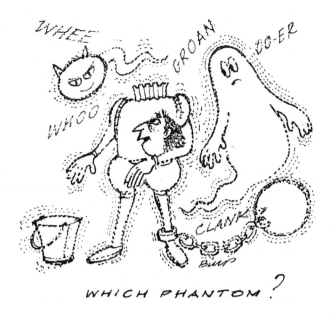

WHICH PHANTOM ?

to the nominated individual, which is retained for reference.

Elsewhere, details of necessary arrangements will be available from the Ministry of Home Affairs or equivalent.

Other radiation work

Any person undertaking work with ionizing radiation (such as use of an X-ray fluoroscopy unit) must demonstrate competence in both radiation protection and the practical procedures to be performed. Using X-ray equipment on patients before becoming proficient could result in administering a higher radiation dose than necessary and should not be permitted. Phantoms can be made available for learning the use of equipment. It is even possible to use a plastic bucket filled with water, and containing radiopaque objects, as a phantom, whilst training.

Note: Whenever demonstrating or testing a piece of fluoroscopy equipment, *never* allow the unattenuated primary X-ray beam to strike the image intensifier face. To do so can permanently damage the unit. A bucket of water or a lead rubber apron makes an ideal attenuator for this purpose.

IRR 85

These regulations were prepared as part of the Health and Safety at Work Act 1974 and therefore are mainly concerned with the safety of staff and visitors. It is this legislation that required hospitals to name controlled and supervised areas, prepare local rules, monitor doses to staff, identify classified workers, and monitor protective equipment such as lead rubber aprons, Geiger counters, etc. This legislation also specifies dose limits for various personnel.

Responsibilities are mainly those incumbent on the *employer* – to provide a healthy and safe workplace, safety training, safety equipment, maintenance of equipment, monitoring, and funding for all these requirements. The *employee* is responsible for his or her own safety as well as for the safety of others in the department. This includes reporting accidents, near-misses and defects in equipment, and proper record-keeping where appropriate.

A *controlled* area is one in which doses from ionizing radiation are likely to exceed three-tenths of any dose limit for employees over 18 years of age.

A *supervised* area is as for controlled area, but with doses likely to exceed one-tenth of any dose limit.

Radiation Protection Committees (RPCs)

These are established by the employer to monitor and discuss radiation safety issues and constituted an important way for different disciplines within the hospital to meet and work together to improve radiation safety. Members are usually RPAs and radiation protection supervisors (RPSs) of the various radiation and radioactive materials user departments; one consultant radiologist, and a representative of the administration of the hospital.

When the HSE inspectors visit a hospital, the first document requested in the X-ray department is the minutes of the RPC. Inability to produce such a document would meet with serious disapproval.

Record-keeping

Without accurate record-keeping, it is impossible to gather details about an incident or examination at a later stage. The guidance notes require that adequate details are kept about every X-ray examination, to enable accurate dosimetric information to be entered into the patient's notes if required. This is clearly impossible unless records exist of screening times and radiographic factors, repeats if any for plain radiography, and the field sizes used in each projection.

Such requests for dose information are usually on female patients who later find themselves to have been pregnant at the time of the examination. In the future, however, we are likely to see investigations of radiation history for patients who are later found to have malignant disease, particularly where they have undergone high-dose investigations such as barium enema, abdominal angiography or computed tomography (see Chapter 7).

Accurate records on the administration and disposal of radioactive materials are vital to ensure patients are given correct doses, as well as for the protection of the environment. Such records also assist the pollution inspectorate to locate and prosecute unscrupulous individuals who may be dispensing and disposing without proper licensing.

In conclusion, accurate dose data for our patients coupled with long-term follow-up will eventually assist the radiology community to reach a more reliable assessment of the risks of low-level X-radiation. The current position is still somewhat speculative. All members of the radiological and radiographic community have an important role to play in ensuring that these data exist.

Dose limits

In the appendix to the IRR 85 are listed the dose limits for workers. These are as follows:

Classified workers

These are the only staff who may receive in excess of three-tenths of a dose limit. Their doses must still be kept as low as reasonably practicable (ALARP). These workers must be kept under careful medical supervision and their radiation dose records kept for 50 years. This category includes persons such as nuclear power station staff, industrial radiographers, and those involved in nuclear reprocessing, but seldom includes hospital staff (the possible exception is those radiologists working extensively in interventional radiology):

- 50 mSv/year: for the whole body.
- 150 mSv/year: for the lens of the eye.
- 500 mSv/year: for individual organs or tissues.
- 13 mSv in any consecutive 3-month period: for the abdomen of a woman of reproductive capacity.
- 10 mSv during the declared term of pregnancy: for the abdomen of a pregnant woman. ICRP 1990 revised this down to 2 mSv.

Note: 1990 recommendations of ICRP have revised the 50 mSv limit. It is now $20 \, \text{mSv} \, \text{y}^{-1}$ averaged over 5 years, with no more than 50 mSv in a single year. At the time of writing this has not yet been legally adopted in the UK.

Non-classified persons

These fall into two categories – radiation workers and any other person.

Radiation workers

Radiation workers are those regularly working with radiation, but who are not likely to approach the three-tenths portion of any dose limit, and who are thus non-classified. (The same dose limits apply to classified employees under 18 years of age.) This category includes radiographers, radiologists and X-ray nursing staff.

Dose limits for these personnel are up to three-tenths of those for classified workers, that is:

- up to 15 mSv/year: for the whole body.
- up to 45 mSv/year: for the lens of the eye.
- up to 150 mSv/year: for individual organs or tissues.

Note: these figures for non-classified radiation workers are not dose limits in the strict sense, but if any non-classified radiation worker comes close to these threshold values, he or she will need to become a classified worker.

Any other person

Any other person covers *visitors* to the X-ray department. This includes people such as the parent of a young patient who may be asked to hold the child for examination; a fetus inside a radiation worker; patients in a waiting area before and after, but not during, their examination. (There are no dose limits for patients whilst undergoing their examinations.) Dose limits for these persons are one-tenth of those for classified workers:

- up to 5 mSv/year: for the whole body. (1 mSv y^{-1} recommended by ICRP in 1990.)
- up to 15 mSv/year: for the lens of the eye.
- up to 50 mSv/year: for individual organs or tissues.

Local rules – radiology department

IRR 85 required every X-ray department to prepare *Local Rules*. This document is the written description of how to comply with the IRR 85 regulations in that department. It must contain a definition and description of the controlled and supervised areas in the department, with plans. There will also be *systems of work* (guidelines on how to be safe in a controlled area) to enable non-classified persons to enter a controlled area, and procedures to restrict access to those areas. In addition the local rules must include contingency plans. These are directions for personnel on how to react in radiation emergencies. Such emergencies include radioactive contamination incidents, overexposure incidents, irradiation of a fetus, and any other untoward occurrence.

Format of local rules

The format is a matter for local decision by the RPS and RPA. It will usually follow these or similar lines:

1. Introduction, with the purpose of the rules.
2. Identities of key personnel with their duties.
3. List of controlled and supervised areas, with plans and descriptions.
4. Systems of work, to enable non-classified workers to enter the controlled area without unwittingly becoming a classified worker (due to exceeding three-tenths of a dose limit!)
5. Operational procedures, or general safety guidelines. These include safety for patients undergoing examination.
6. Contingency plans; emergency action plans.
7. An appendix of useful information, and telephone numbers of key personnel.

Emergencies

In an emergency you may need to contact the RPA and RPS. You may also need to consult the local rules for emergency contingency plans (see Chapters 7 and 9 for more information). Do not panic. It is very unlikely that an overexposure from diagnostic X-ray equipment has caused any serious injury to your patient or yourself.

11

Reduction of radiation doses to staff

Introduction

We could reduce our radiation doses by becoming journalists instead. Alternatively, we can adopt sensible measures such as those cited below, and doses can be reduced accordingly. Additionally, there are various features of departmental design, construction and accessories which contribute to lowering staff doses. We must avoid the pollution of our genetic material by striving for the lowest possible radiation doses.

Radiation doses received by diagnostic radiographers and radiologists

These are extremely low, of the order of 2.0 mSv or less per year whole body dose (in addition to background dose). Most are due to fluoroscopy and mobile radiography duties.

Doses received by staff in radiotherapy departments

These are often lower than the 2.0 mSv received by diagnostic radiographers due to the shielding from cosmic radiation afforded by the thick protective concrete walls of most radiotherapy departments.

Personal monitoring requirements

The practice of personal monitoring has no direct effect on staff doses. Monitoring of personal doses is only obligatory for classified workers (see Chapter 10 for dose limits and definitions of this category). For non-classified radiation workers, there are less stringent requirements: these are to monitor the environment and a representative sample of the staff. The radiation records for non-classified radiation workers must be kept for just 2 years after recording, whereas those for classified workers must be kept for 50 years. An authorized (by the Health and Safety Executive) or approved dosimetry laboratory must be used when doses to classified workers are to be measured.

Personal monitoring devices

Monitoring will indicate poor protection practice, and help to determine the doses received during accidents. The various devices available are described below.

Film badges

A double-emulsion photographic film, mounted in a holder, is worn to record the doses received. The holder consists of filters of different thicknesses and materials and enables the monitoring service to determine information on the energy and type of radiation received by the wearer.

The filters are:

- Lead/tin (200 keV to 2 MeV photons).
- Lead/cadmium (slow neutrons).
- Dural (an aluminium/copper alloy).
- Thin and thick plastic (diagnostic-range X-rays).

Each batch of film requires calibration, using a radioactive source (e.g. caesium 137). Calibration badges in their holders receive a known exposure varied in time or distance from the source (Fig. 11.1).

Advantages

Film badges are cheap, and allow much information on the type of radiation responsible for the exposure. If a dose is due to radioactive materials spill, it will show up as spots on the film.

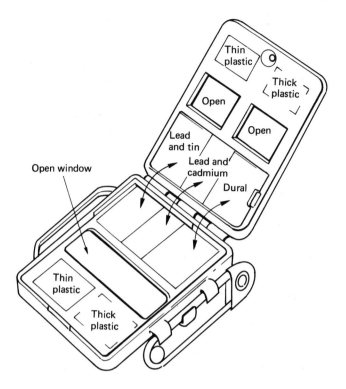

Fig. 11.1 Badge holder for monitoring radiation.

An image of a rib or other body part indicates that the wearer was in the primary beam. Recording range is wide due to the presence of both a fast and a slow emulsion. If the fast emulsion is blackened, it can be stripped away and the slow one used alone, recording over a wider range of doses.

Disadvantages

Threshold is high at 0.2 mSv. Film badges usually need to be changed monthly, which is inaccurate for low doses, and demanding on administrative effort. Holders are expensive. Filters can be misplaced, giving inaccurate results. Storage conditions can affect results.

Thermoluminescent dosimeters

These consist of polytetrafluorethylene (PTFE) wafers or discs which are impregnated with a thermoluminescent material. Such materials store the energy of any incident ionizing radiation photon by having electrons temporarily held in electron traps at higher than normal energy bands. When the radiation dosage is to be measured, the wafer is heated and the electrons are released from the traps. Light is given off; its quantity is proportional to the amount of incident ionizing radiation absorbed by the wafer.

There are several materials commonly used for this purpose. Calcium sulphate and lithium fluoride are two examples. The calcium type is extremely sensitive to low energy (scattered) radiation; the lithium type has a long-proven track record for reliability, and both can be reused repeatedly.

Doses to staff during angiography

Doses to the patient and staff for cine-angiography and interventional radiology are very high. Staff thus receive appreciable doses and operator and scrub assistant should wear 0.35 mm lead-equivalent aprons during angiography procedures. Also the operator should attempt to stand back by at least 30 cm during exposures (Balver et al. 1978).

In cineradiography there are considerable advantages in using pulsed-output, grid control tubes. The tube is only energized when the film is still – for 6 ms for every image. Radiation-on time is precisely synchronized with film position, saving patient and staff dose as well as wear and tear on equipment (Forster, 1985).

One method to reduce eye dose involves the use of a lead glass screen suspended from the ceiling between the patient and operator or scrub nurse (American Journal of Radiology, 1979). This can reduce eye doses by up to 35% of former level. Protective lead glasses may be uncomfortable and one design will not fit all head shapes. As a general rule, personal protective equipment is not the first line of approach when a hazard requiring its use is a frequent occurrence.

Eye doses can be measured approximately at the neck, ideally

Table 11.1 DOSES IN mSv/CASE FOR CINE
CARDIAC ANGIOGRAPHY (R. CONNETT
HDCR MODULE F PROJECT 1987)

Staff and body organ	Dose
Cardiologist	
Eye	0.174
Gonad	0.039
Radiologist	
Eye	0.065
Gonad	< 0.05
Scrub assistant	
Eye	0.069
Gonad	0.019
Nurse	
Eye	0.291
Gonad	0.007
Cardiac technician	
Eye	0.074
Gonad	< 0.05
Radiographer	
Eye	0.024
Gonad	< 0.05

using a different type of badge for outside and inside the apron to avoid confusion.

The figures shown in Table 11.1 were considerably reduced in the second period of monitoring; perhaps staff became more careful with their safety. Based on the results of the research quoted, the cardiologist could perform up to 280 such cases per year without needing to become classified workers (about 5 cases per week). For other staff, except nurses, considerably more cases could be performed without the need for them to become classified workers.

Finger dosimetry results

- 0.155 mSv/case for a cardiologist.
- 0.130 mSv/case for a radiologist.

Interestingly, the body and eye doses for radiologists were approximatly one-third of those for cardiologists, but the finger

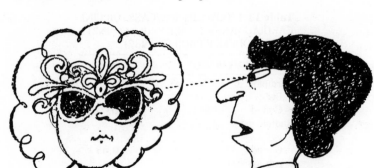

' NOT QUITE WHAT WE HAD IN MIND DOCTOR !

doses were almost the same. The differences may be due to one or more of the following:

1. Do cardiologists take the more difficult cases?
2. Are radiologists more careful to protect themselves?
3. The fingers may be better protected by the brachial approach favoured by cardiologists, rather than the femoral approach favoured by radiologists.
4. A combination of all three is likely. It is however interesting to see the improvement later in the study. Judging by the similarity in finger doses, it suggests that the difficult cases are not requiring a more lengthy catheter manipulation.

Nursing staff receive surprisingly high eye doses. The nurse's position is usually at the head of the patient. These members of staff thus get no benefit from the protective apron, explorator etc. The nurse frequently leans forward to comfort the patient, giving him- or herself a higher dose.

It is a duty of the radiographer to protect and advise nursing staff on how best to protect themselves, particularly for eye doses.

Eye protection during interventional radiology

Lead glass spectacles should be made available for all personnel, especially nursing staff, who often are involved in a larger proportion of the cases than other professionals. These spectacles are available for as little as the price of a pair of designer sunglasses. For those who wear glasses, photochromatic glass lenses offer greater protection than other types of eyewear. Prescription lead spectacles are an option for frequent users, and are available to order from protective equipment manufacturers. Lateral protection is particularly important for the radiologist, whose eyes are trained on the television monitor whilst screening, and thus he or she receives radiation from the sides.

Dose reduction during computed tomography

When injecting a dose of contrast medium for an enhanced study, the radiologist should avoid standing close to the patient during the scan. The high kilovoltages employed for this modality produce high keV sideways scatter, and the radiologist positioned nearby will consequently receive a high dose. An autoinjector can be used, but a better method is to use extension tubes to increase the distance, and flush through with saline afterwards (Hawkins and Turner, 1989).

Lead rubber aprons

Lead rubber aprons are available in various different designs and lead equivalents, for example, 0.35 or 0.5 mm on the front only, for interventional work. It is advisable to cover the sternum and shoulders completely to reduce red bone marrow dose. Alternatively use thyroid collars, and longer-length aprons to cover the femora. Conventional lead rubber apron designs cover approximately 73% of the red bone marrow. An apron which covers the sternum, thyroid, lower third of the cervical spine and humeral heads shields 84% of the red bone marrow. This is at marginal extra cost, and minimal loss of comfort (Boothroyd and Russell, 1987).

Hand protection

Lead rubber gloves are a vital part of the protective equipment. They are usually of 0.5 mm lead-equivalent, and resemble a gauntlet in design. Other types may also be useful, for example an open-palm design can be more practical for holding a child's hands during radiography, or for the orthopaedic surgeon whilst manipulating for stress views. Lead rubber sterilizable gloves have become available. These offer a little protection from scatter and none from primary radiation. They can give staff a false sense of security, and as such are of questionable value. Fine tube manipulation and holding of children are impossible with such gloves.

Case study

During safety training, an orthopaedic surgeon asked: 'How can I possibly manipulate a fracture without getting my hands in the primary beam?' A reply was not necessary, since another orthopaedic surgeon from the audience replied that it was absolutely possible, and failing to do so set a bad example to junior staff. He went on to say that he manipulated the part, then removed his hands and viewed the alignment under X-ray control. This was a powerful message coming from a fellow professional doing the same work.

This case study is a graphic example of how training courses are far more useful than book-based study, and the requirement for 'core of knowledge' courses in the UK has been an extremely useful development.

Fluoroscopy dose reduction to staff

In undercouch screening equipment, the X-ray tube is installed beneath the X-ray table, and the image intensifier (or explorator) moves around above the patient, coupled to the tube beneath. This arrangement reduces staff doses compared with overcouch screening (tube above, image intensifier below patient).

Overcouch screening is usually designed as a remote-control facility, which is undesirable in terms of patient care and attention. Full co-operation when a remote control system is in use requires a thorough explanation before commencing, and a rehearsal of positioning, which lengthens the examination. The dose to the patient with overcouch screening (due to the longer focus patient distance) can be reduced by up to 50% compared with the undercouch alternative.

Overcouch screening units should never be used for interventional radiology, unless lead protective equipment is installed about the tubehead. This can compromise a sterile field, but without it there is inadequate protection for personnel who remain in the room.

Paediatric fluoroscopy

For paediatric departments, however, a different priority exists. Every case involves irradiation of an individual of childbearing capacity. The genetically significant dose is far higher, and staff cease to be the critical group for radiation dose. Peak kilovoltage is lower than for adult work and thus staff doses are reduced. In the examination of children, the use of overcouch fluoroscopy could replace undercouch fluoroscopy, even for interventional work, achieving large savings in patient dose.

Training and specialization

Adequate training, including work such as practice on a dummy aorta, watching others perform the procedure several times, and visiting specialist centres, is vital in ensuring doses are kept as low as reasonably achievable.

The complicated nature of many aspects of radiography or radiology demands highly skilled staff. Specialization of radiology staff ensures high standards of practice, familiarity with equipment and techniques, motivation, and a total familiarity with the respective roles of each member of the team.

Protection of staff

Due to beam hardening within the patient, scattered radiation is rather more penetrating than we might care to imagine. Much of the data previously available on beam transmission referred to narrow beam measurements which do not really mirror the conditions in radiographic practice where a broad beam situation always exists.

Table 11.2 PERCENTAGE OF BROAD BEAM TRANSMISSION AT DIFFERENT KILOVOLTAGE SELECTIONS

Generating voltage	Transmission of 90° scatter (0.25 mm Pb apron)	As a pecentage of unshielded dose (0.35 mm Pb apron)
50	0.92%	0.23%
60	1.70%	0.62%
70	3.3%	1.5%
80	4.4%	2.1%
90	5.8%	2.8%
100	8.6%	4.6%
110	12%	6.6%
120	15%	8.6%

Table 11.3 RED BONE MARROW DISTRIBUTION IN THE ADULT JAPANESE POPULATION

Part of the body	Percentage red bone marrow
Humerus	3.6%
Femora	14.4%
Ilium	22.2%
Ribs	13.6%
Sacrum	8.6%
Lumbar spine	11.2%
Thoracic spine	13.2%
Skull	7.2%
Cervical spine	2.9%
Clavicle	0.7%
Mandible	0.5%
Scapula	2.2%

(from Nishizawa et al. British Journal of Radiology Jan. 1991).

The difference in bone marrow distribution between the Japanese and other racial groups is not believed to be significant.

From the data given in Table 11.2 there appears to be a very strong case for 0.35 mm lead-equivalent aprons particularly at higher kilovoltages where savings are very large. For barium enemas, the larger element of overcouch radiography during the examination allows the wearer to remove the apron between cases, reducing back fatigue.

Table 11.3 illustrates the whereabouts of red bone marrow in

Table 11.4 ALTERNATIVES TO LEAD PLY

Material	Density (kg/m³)	Thickness (mm)	Lead equivalents (mm)	
			70/5 kV$_p$	150 kV$_p$
Barytes plaster	2110	12.7	1.1	0.9
Breeze blocks	1270	126	0.8	0.7
Brick				
Yellow	1600	114	0.9	0.9
Red	1850	128	1.2	1.05
Concrete				
Solid	2350	75	0.9	0.9
Block	1660	122	1.12	0.92
Aerated	850	75	$\simeq 0.19$	0.22
Steel sheet	7900	5	0.9	0.43

(HPA report 41: Notes on building materials and references on shielding data for use below 300 kV$_p$, 1984)

adults, indicating where the greatest protection priorities may lie. Approximately 80% of the red bone marrow is under a conventional lead rubber apron, but one can save as much as 6% more by wearing a thyroid collar.

Building materials

In order to protect staff and patients from radiation, walls and protective screens must provide adequate shielding. Lead ply is usually the first material considered, but it is costly and only available from specialist companies. There are however a number of extremely effective alternatives. The suitability of each depends on the application required. Always consult the radiation protection adviser (RPA) at the planning stage. Adding shielding later is costly and may require redecoration and additional down time.

Walls and doors

Because of the tendency for lead to 'creep', it cannot be fixed to a wall as sheet lead metal, but must be first sandwiched between two sheets of plywood and glued securely. Any fixings, such as nails or screws, must be plugged with lead to preserve the protective integrity of the panel or door. Alternatives to lead ply are given in Table 11.4. As can be seen, a number of practical alternatives to lead ply exist for use on wall shielding. Older, sturdily built premises may not require additional shielding. The protective qualities must always be verified by testing, because of the variations in building materials and methods.

Floors and ceilings

Where an X-ray unit is operated above or below an inhabited area, the floor of the room in use or the floor of the room above may need shielding to protect those below or above. One inexpensive option to protect persons in the room above is to roll a thick sheet of builders' lead over the floor, covered with hardboard, then with normal floor-covering. It is not practical to apply Barytes plaster to a ceiling when the protection can be more conveniently placed on to the floor of the room above. Always consult the RPA.

How thick does the shielding need to be?

This question can only be answered by the RPA. In order to make an informed decision, he or she will require the following estimated information:

- Likely workload in mA min/day (total mA/day divided by 60).
- Relative proportions of maximum kilovoltage to be used.
- Relative proportions of vertical (up) beam work, if any.
- Relative proportions of horizontal beam work and in which directions.
- Nature and occupancy of rooms above, below, adjacent.

Armed with this information, the RPA will then calculate the radiation levels likely to be incident on the walls, floor, ceilings, protective console screen, doors and windows of the room. Measurements may also be required of the protective properties of building materials used in the construction of the X-ray room. Calculations will then be made to ascertain the radiation shielding required (with a comfort margin to allow for an increase over the projected workload) to reduce the incident radiation to a safe level for people on the other side.

For a general X-ray room the protection calculations may be complicated. Any point in the room may receive primary radiation, partially attenuated primary radiation, and scattered radiation depending on beam directions. The energy of the radiation will vary from a few tens of keV to 150 keV (depending upon whether it is primary or scattered in origin). The wall behind a chest stand or vertical bucky will always require additional shielding, as will the wall adjacent to the X-ray table during horizontal beam work. Local rules may need to incorporate a forbidden beam direction if the capacity for accidental irradiation exists.

Whenever new techniques are to be introduced which involve new positions, directions or energies of the primary beam, the RPA must be informed. The protective equipment or shielding in the room may need to be reviewed.

Once a new room or installation is on line, environmental monitoring (usually employing personal monitoring dosimeters) will be required to verify the adequacy of the protective shielding in the room. Protective lead ply panels have occasionally been found to be leadless on close examination.

Conclusion

This chapter has given an overview of the measures of dose reduction for staff. Some of these measures are extremely costly, and will require a properly presented case to secure the necessary funding. The provision of protective equipment is most important for techniques which are performed frequently, especially where a small number of staff are particularly at risk.

Sadly, protective equipment is easily misplaced, or disappears when personnel move to other hospitals. To minimize this problem, a nominated individual (plus a deputy to cover holidays and sickness) should act as custodian, rather like a librarian, and keep the lead goggles and thyroid collars in an accessible but secure place.

12

Nuclear medicine

This chapter covers techniques for general dose reduction in a small nuclear medicine department. There are also specific points for the protection of children, the baby of a nursing mother, and children of a patient undergoing examination. Dose limitation for the staff in the nuclear medicine department is considered, as well as those elsewhere in the hospital who may deal with radioactive patients.

Note: The points below are for guidance only. Personnel involved in a nuclear medicine facility *must* consult the radiation protection adviser (RPA) before commencing the service. Policy reflecting expert local clinical and radiological protection opinion must be formulated. There is a legal requirement on the employer to appoint and consult an RPA.

Departmental design

The first step in ensuring safety in a nuclear medicine department is in the proper design of that area. The RPA should be consulted at the drawing-board stage. The layout of the department is extremely important. The ability to cordon off the whole area in the event of a contamination incident is crucial. If there remains a need for people to wander through, spreading the contamination, a major incident could develop.

There must be adequate space to allow the best use to be made of inverse square law protection. There should be separate areas for the preparation and storage of radioactive materials, and comfortable waiting areas for the patients. An area is required to store radioactive waste, away from camera and patients.

The room where injections are administered must be well away from the gamma camera or the radioactivity could affect the images. Emergency decontamination facilities are an important requirement. The necessary office space must not be too close to where radioactive materials are used and stored, or staff doses will be higher than necessary.

Minimum facilities required, assuming no on-site radiopharmacy

1. An adequate waiting area to allow patients to wait comfortably, but not so close to each other that they undergo mutual irradiation.
2. A separate radionuclide preparation room with lead protective vials, screens, containers and personal protective equipment to keep dose rates low and protect staff from contamination.
3. A separate injection room with an adequate supply of syringe shields, which can reduce finger pulp doses by 75%.
4. A large gamma camera room with an adequate area to store collimators and computers, in which trolleys can be turned around and which is pleasant and airy.
5. Quality assurance equipment: a regularly replaced flood source is required to check for failed photomultiplier tubes before every scan. A well counter calibration source is needed to check injection doses. Other articles of test equipment such as resolution grids can be shared between neighbouring centres in a locality.
6. Emergency equipment: decontamination kit, emergency shower facilities, contamination monitor (with recent calibration), store for radioactive waste, thorough contingency plans detailing how to deal with any emergency situation.

Walls, worktops and flooring

Wherever radioactive materials are handled the surfaces should be easily decontaminated, i.e. sealed worktops, impervious flooring coved up the walls, with a shiny surface (however, avoid slip hazards). Sealed sinks must be provided with *elbow-control* taps, to avoid hands passing contamination on to taps then on to others. Good-pressure water flow which does not spray will enable the speedy dilution of disposed liquids and avoid droplets contaminating passing staff. Ideally the water should be artifici-

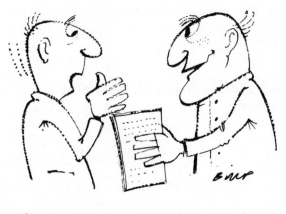

' THIS IS A VERY GLOWING
REPORT DOCTOR ! '

ally softened to avoid limescale build-up. Hard water allows adherence of heavy radioactive atoms and causes contamination to build up around the plug hole area and in the trap. Where elbow taps have not been provided, as an interim measure, polythene bags can be fixed over the tap handles; these bags can easily be discarded if they do become contaminated. Large traps are not advisable and the plumbing should be easily accessible for repairs, maintenance and contamination checks. Sinks used for radioactive waste disposal must be labelled as such and listed in the Local Rules. The drain runs from these sinks should go out directly to the foul drains, to avoid risk of radioactive liquid coming up in a sink elsewhere in the building in a blockage scenario. The manhole covers for such drains should be painted yellow to alert maintenance staff to the possible hazard of radioactive contamination.

Always seek advice from the RPA when a laboratory is being planned, refurbished or modified. This can save costly modifications later.

General principles

Three principles will help keep staff doses ALARA (as low as reasonably achievable): time, distance and shielding.

Time

Work efficiently and *keep clear of the radioactive area when your presence there is unnecessary.*

Desks and chairs, telephones and magazines should never be placed in radioactive materials areas as they encourage personnel to linger.

Remove all contaminated articles to a safe, shielded disposal area – leaving them lying around simply increases the ambient radiation dose levels, heightening the risk of personnel contamination and raising the possibility of airborne contamination.

Once a patient has received a radioactive dose by whatever route, that person becomes a radioactive source. A bone scan patient can impart a dose of 20 μSv/h at 0.5 m. This is equivalent to a time average dose rate of 13 μSv/h, and in excess of the 7.5 μSv/h controlled area threshold. Two such patients in the waiting area require designation of a controlled area.

Distance

Distance yourself from radioactive sources. The inverse square law will usefully protect staff. One hospital converted an entire ward to become the nuclear medicine department. Because of the large distance between the operator, the camera and the radioactive materials storage position, no heavy shielding was required and the whole department had a light, airy atmosphere. Doubling the distance from the source reduces the dose rate by a factor of four.

In the waiting area, it is far more pleasant for patients to be separated from each other by permanently fixed pots of plants and coffee tables, than to be ordered to keep away from each other by frightening warning notices.

Being radioactive is a thoroughly unpleasant experience for our patients. They associate their situation with atomic bombs and nuclear power stations. Thorough explanations are extremely important but the sensitivities of already unwell patients must be considered at every stage. Most important is to assure them that they are only very slightly radioactive, and that it is shortlived.

Shielding

The use of properly designed lead shields for vials and tungsten or lead glass syringe shields can considerably reduce staff doses. Use long-handled forceps with non-slip rubber-covered grips and specially designed carrying handles to keep radioactive sources well away from the operator's fingers and minimize finger pulp doses. Use a syringe one size larger than necessary – this keeps fingers further from the source. Westminster Hospital nuclear medicine department have designed an excellent and inexpensive mechanical injector which is most effective.

Lead rubber aprons are of *no use whatsoever* to personnel in nuclear medicine. Isotopes which are suitable for the gamma camera produce highly energetic gamma radiation, which will pass through lead rubber as if it were soft butter. Wearing a lead apron will slow you down in your work, increasing your dose. *Don't wear them.*

Radioactive waste

Radioactive waste should also be treated as hazardous and stored in shielded bins, to decay, or be incinerated where appropriate.

Nuclear medicine patients requiring other studies

In order to satisfy the ALARA principle, nuclear medicine patients who require other studies, such as skeletal survey, should not have the radiographs taken after the radionuclide injection has been given. This causes the patient to become a radioactive source and consequently gives a radiation dose to the examining radiographer that he or she need not receive. Whilst at first sight it may appear more efficient to inject the patient, then X-ray, then scan, from a clinical viewpoint this is inadvisable. Bone changes reveal themselves far sooner on a bone scan than on a radiographic study. Consequently, 'hot spots' found on the bone scan can be followed up by coned views of the regions of concern rather than doing a generalized survey. If it is vital that they be performed on the same day as the bone scan, and cannot be scheduled before the injection is given, then the patient should be radiographed after the bone scan has been completed, allowing the radioactivity to have decayed considerably. In many cases the useful scan results may completely nullify the requirement for a skeletal survey, which is time-consuming, costly and, worst of all, the various positions required may be thoroughly unpleasant for a patient who is already in pain.

Contamination

Personnel in nuclear medicine departments are at far greater risk from internal radioactive contamination than from external radiation doses. In order to protect themselves, high standards of personal hygiene are necessary. Waterproof aprons and double latex gloves (PVC gloves allow technetium and iodine to penetrate) are vital. Fabric treatment to make white coats water-repellent are also beneficial.

The most important action however is regular washing of hands before eating, drinking, smoking, *visiting the toilet*, applying make-up and going for breaks. Use the contamination monitor to check hands and clothing. If stubborn contamination remains on hands after washing, a useful technique is to don polythene gloves and allow sweating to remove the contamination from inside outwards.

Never eat, drink or apply cosmetics in the nuclear medicine department. Use disposable paper tissues to blow the nose, discarding them immediately after use. Never use linen or cotton handkerchiefs which can hold contamination and irradiate the person from inside the pockets. See local rules.

Protection of the patient

A very high-quality examination will give the most accurate diagnosis and this must be the aim in every case, avoiding the need for a repeat with extra radiation dose. The minimum activity necessary for good results is most important. All these points are indicated in the *Notes for Guidance on the Administration of Radioactive Substances to Persons for the Purposes of Diagnosis, Treatment or Research*. (Available free of charge from the ARSAC secretariat at the Department of Health see Addresses in Appendix.)

Table 12.1 CALCULATION OF DOSE ACCORDING TO CHILDREN'S BODY WEIGHT AND SURFACE AREA

	Body weight	Surface area
For a newborn		
Divide adult dose by	17	7
For a 1-year-old		
Divide adult dose by	6	3
For a 5-year-old		
Divide adult dose by	3.3	2.3
For a 10-year-old		
Divide adult dose by	2	1.7

Quoted figures apply to those studies based on body weight and surface area. For a 15-year-old divide by 1.1.
To calculate patient surface area in m^2: 0.14 (body weight in kg)$^{2/3}$.

Plan the day to ensure adequate time for good scans.

All patients should be encouraged to drink plenty on the day of their scan, and to empty the bladder frequently. This will avoid high radiation doses to the gonads or pelvic bone marrow.

Nuclear medicine studies on children

Where children are examined, the activity administered must be carefully calculated acording to data contained in the Guidance Notes.

One method to determine the activity to be administered is given in Table 12.1.

Carefully ascertain if the mother of a young child undergoing the study is pregnant and advise accordingly. Children may need admitting to hospital to protect an unborn sibling.

Young patients should be advised to drink plenty and frequently. This will encourage them to empty the bladder often (in a baby a wet nappy should be changed frequently) to avoid irradiating the gonads and bone marrow in the pelvis from a 'hot' bladder. A full bladder can also obscure pelvic pathology, e.g. in the sacrum or pubis, or an ectopic phaeochromocytoma. Beware of artefacts from urine spots on underwear.

Children have a higher metabolic rate and may need to be scanned earlier than adults following injection for the same examination. Seek expert local advice.

Training

Nuclear medicine is an exacting procedure and should only be practised by properly trained and supervised personnel. The College of Radiographers in the UK offers an excellent diploma course in nuclear medicine, which is recognized worldwide.

The pregnant patient

Ideally pregnant patients are not examined using radioactive materials but where this is vital for patient management, dose limitation must be considered a priority.

- Modify the study: e.g. perfusion only for lung study.
- Reduce the dose given to the minimum possible, but not so low as to compromise results.
- Choose a radiopharmaceutical with a short biological half-life – one that is rapidly cleared from the body. (Consult the RPA and where necessary adjust timing of study.)
- Segregate the pregnant patient from other patients to avoid her receiving a dose from them.

The breast-feeding mother

Note: Some women breast-feed babies to beyond the age of 2 years. Take extra care with ethnic minority mothers, where this is more common.

There are two sources of radiation dose to the baby of a breast-feeding mother – direct contact with the mother's body, and ingestion of radiopharmaceutical from the breast milk. A 1991 court ruling in the UK awarded a sizeable compensation to a mother who had not been warned to cease feeding her baby following a radioactive iodine examination.

Suggest reduced contact for 24 h, if it is a technetium study. Offer admission to the patient, if she feels it will help her to reduce contact with the baby.

To keep the dose to below a sensible limit (corrected for body weight), radiopharmaceuticals can be divided into three groups:

1. There is no need to interrupt feeding, e.g. ^{99m}Tc diethylenetri-aminepentaacetic acid, HDP, DMSA, MDP, ^{111}I leucocytes.
2. Interrupt for 24 h, express and discard the milk, e.g. ^{99m}Tc pertechnetate, ^{99m}Tc erythrocytes, EDTA (MAA interrupt 9 hours).
3. Completely discontinue, e.g. ^{67}Ga citrate, ^{131}Iodide.

Note: this guidance applies to mature breast milk, *not* colostrum.

For compounds with low breast milk excretion, we can further reduce the dose by advising the mother to feed her baby immediately before administration of the dose.

The first feed (about 4 h after administration) is expressed and discarded, then feeding is resumed normally. If doubts remain, ask the mother to express the milk, count in a counter and make an informed decision at that point. Always consult the RPA in such cases.

Observation of these measures will help to satisfy the ALARA principle for these patients (Smith 1986).

For further guidance see IPSM Report 63. *Radiation Protection in Nuclear Medicine and Pathology* (1991).

Appendix

Action in case of incontinent patient accident on the ward following a radioactive material investigation

Note: Guidelines should be drawn up in advance as part of the contingency plans in the local rules. Copies should be sent to all wards from which nuclear medicine scan patients may be referred. Incontinent patients should be catheterized before undergoing any nuclear medicine procedure.

Emergency action following an incontinent patient incident

You have probably turned to this page in panic with the ward on the phone at 11.00 p.m. one evening whilst on call. If nuclear medicine personnel are not available, ask the switchboard to contact the RPS if possible. Then:

- Advise the nurse in charge to clear the area of non-essential staff, visitors and patients.
- Don two pairs of *latex* gloves, a waterproof apron and over-shoes.

Note: A pregnant member of staff should not perform this duty.

- Mop up any floor contamination with incontinence pads.
- Remove the patient's clothing and bed linen and double bag. Wash down the mattress with a disinfectant using *disposable* cleaning cloths. Treat contaminated articles and body fluids as if they were a biohazard. Double bag and retain.
- Store all double-bagged linen and disposables in a remote secure section of the ward, allowing radioactive decay to reduce the hazard. Contact the nuclear medicine staff in the morning for advice before disposing of wastes or sending articles to the laundry.
- Record all details of the incident for a formal report. This will be required so that action can be taken to avoid a repeat occurrence.

13
Non-ionizing radiation

Non-ionizing radiation safety

As technology progresses, new developments are quickly adapted for use in medicine. This chapter is a brief outline of the possible risks to patients and staff from these technologies, and how to reduce these risks. For a more thorough understanding, consult the listed references. The employer should appoint an expert advisor, consult the RPA if in doubt.

Ultrasound

The use of sound waves to image the fetus or internal organs has done much to reduce the amount of ionizing radiation used for such investigations. Many fetal abnormalities are now detected early enough for a safe termination, or so that preparation can be made for prompt action immediately after delivery. Ultrasound scanning has replaced a number of invasive diagnostic investigations and increased the speed of diagnosis for many patients.

There are known to be several potentially hazardous effects due to ultrasound, but **these have not** been recorded at the energy levels used for diagnosis. Nevertheless, the amount of ultrasound energy input needs to be carefully restricted, especially for Doppler studies near to the gonads and the fetus *in utero*. The hazardous effects can be described as follows.

Possible damage due to physical effects

1. Heat production – heat can 'cook' or denature proteins. Ultrasound waves can intensify the cell-killing effects of heat

and of cytotoxic drugs, especially if intensity exceeds 3 W/cm^2, and frequency is at 3 MHz or above.

2. At peaks and troughs of sound waves, cells can be pressed together; red blood cells can damage vessel walls. This is seen if intensity exceeds 1 W/cm^2.

3. Platelets can undergo aggregation (clumping together). Damage is seen if intensities exceed 0.2 W/cm^2 at 1 MHz for 5 min.

4. Streaming – this is rather like convection currents in a heated saucepan of water, and is of unknown consequence in the embryo.

5. Cavitation effects – bubbles form and burst. The threshold intensity is higher at higher frequencies. Threshold is about 1 W/cm^2 at 1 MHz. The formation and bursting of gas bubbles in tissue are believed to cause various potentially harmful consequences, such as free radical (e.g. hydrogen peroxide) formation, mechanical erosion of solids, disruption of long chain molecules, emulsification of mixtures and aerosol formation. These may be easier to produce in a test-tube than in a person due to the greater quantity of dissolved gases in test-tubes.

Ultrasound is also used in physiotherapy departments for the treatment of joint and muscle injury. It is known to stimulate collagen synthesis and accelerate tissue healing. The power levels are far higher in physiotherapy than those used in imaging – 0.1–0.4 W/cm^2, whereas for imaging 0.005–0.01 W/cm^2 is used. (This may be higher for Doppler (blood flow imaging), but pulsed so overall energy input is below damage threshold.)

The following practical guidance points will help improve safety: prudence is advised for imaging M-mode or colour Doppler. There is no evidence to preclude a diagnostic study which could result in useful diagnostic information. It is vital to ensure output is kept as low as reasonably practicable and regularly monitored. The range of intensities used by different centres varies enormously – up to 40 times between minimum and maximum for the same type of scan.

Practical guidance for the safe use of diagnostic ultrasound scanners

The sonographer should at all times:

1. Keep output to the minimum necessary for the clinical results required.
2. Minimize time that the transducer is in contact with skin surface; keep it moving, and not in the same place for long periods.
3. Obtain exposure information from supplier or local medical physics service.
4. Be aware of the effects of the control settings on exposure to the patient.
5. Check the maximum temperature that can be reached by the transducer, particularly when used for intracavitary work.

For pulsed Doppler ultrasound, *greater caution is necessary*. In addition to the above:

1. Take particular care in obstetric applications.
2. Keep total acoustic power to a minimum.
3. Keep pulse amplitude to a minimum.
4. Minimize exposure of tissue–bone interfaces.
5. Exercise particular caution if the patient has an elevated body temperature, and for work with babies and children.

(*The Safe Use of Diagnostic Ultrasound*, The British Medical Ultrasound Society, Published by the British Institute of Radiology, 1991.)

The following effects have been induced using *high-intensity* ultrasound: delayed reflex development, altered emotional behaviour, and splenomegaly in rats; fetal abnormality, reduced birth weight, depressed immune response and sarcoma cell induction in mice.

Maximum safe levels

Fetal Doppler, B-mode, real time: $10 \, \text{mW/cm}^2$.
M-mode: $40 \, \text{mW/cm}^2$.
A-mode: $100 \, \text{mW/cm}^2$.

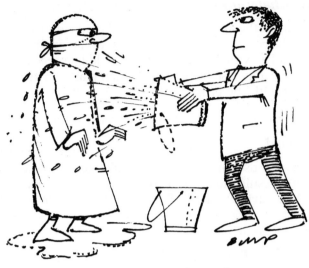

··· *AND DAMPEN FABRIC* ··

Lasers

The word *laser* comes from *l*ight *a*mplification by *s*timulated *e*mission of *r*adiation. The input energy is transformed into an intense beam of light, all of one wavelength.

The hazards to staff and patients during the use of medical lasers are as follows.

Eye damage

This may be to retina or cornea depending on wavelength. Always use protective eyewear, and moist swabs for the patient. Check that the eyewear used is appropriate for the wavelengths employed. Seek advice from the laser protection adviser.

Skin damage

Skin damage includes burns and depigmentation. Always wear long-sleeved theatre gowns and dampen fabric.

Smoke inhalation

Depending on the application, tissue ablation can result in heavy smoke or aerosol, from which there may be an infection risk. Proper smoke extraction apparatus should be used with a laser. Toxic fumes may also be produced when plastic instruments are in contact with the beam.

Fire hazard

Sterile drapes used near the surgery site need to be damp, or a fire hazard results. Keep fire extinguishers and blankets close at hand. Seek advice from the fire officer or local fire brigade.

Anaesthetic gases explosion

If laser procedure is to take place in or near the mouth during a general anaesthetic, laser-proof anaesthetic tubing *must* be used. The laser beam could burn through the tubing otherwise and ignite gases.

Rectal surgery

The rectum should be packed with moist swabs to avoid methane gas explosions from the patient breaking wind. A low-residue diet and exercise prior to the procedure are also beneficial in reducing this hazard.

Quality assurance

The laser should be regularly checked for proper performance. If a visible aiming beam is used with an invisible cutting beam, the alignment should be checked; a wooden spoon is an excellent test tool. Draw circles on it. Fire the beam to check alignment; this is a pass/fail test. Seek guidance from the laser protection adviser (or radiation protection adviser). Power levels require regular verification with calibrated test instruments.

Medical uses

In radiology pulsed dye lasers are used in laser angioplasty. In gynaecology, a carbon dioxide laser is used for resection of cervical precancers. It can also be used for haemorrhoidectomies, oral surgery, and tumour resection, especially for recurrent oesophageal and rectal types, and otherwise inoperable bronchial carcinomas. There is fast healing, little tissue swelling and reduced pain and blood loss.

Local rules are always required and are prepared by the laser protection adviser and laser protection supervisor. Ask to see these. They usually make various provisos, such as illuminated 'in use' signs, and name a key holder, who releases the key only to named individuals.

See for reference: Medical Laser Safety. IPSM Report 48. Institute of Physical Science in Medicine.

Ultraviolet radiation

This is used in the treatment of psoriasis, and for jaundice in the newborn. It is usually under the control of the dermatology department. Ultraviolet radiation can cause eye and skin damage. It is difficult to measure output without specialist equipment. The environment needs proper supervision, and staff require safety training. Safety clothing may be needed for staff. Seek advice from the radiation protection adviser. An additional outside expert may need to be consulted.

Microwave radiation (e.g. diathermy)

The exposure limit in the UK is $10 \, \text{mW/cm}^2$. (Limits are much lower in the former Soviet Union.) Microwave radiation is a hazard to the eye, with risk of cataract formation; to the developing fetus and the testes, due to vulnerability and the inability to dissipate heat. It can also cause headaches, nausea and psychological symptoms.

Wire mesh or thin metal foil completely protects the operator, hence mesh eye protection, as in the door linings of microwave ovens, is worn. Inexpensive meters are now available for safety monitoring.

Diathermy uses 26.5 MHz microwaves. Microwaves ovens employ 2450 MHz waves. Diathermy waves are highly penetrating and can readily heat a human torso.

Magnetic resonance imaging (MRI)

In MRI a powerful, uniform magnetic field is produced and maintained inside a patient tunnel. (The field strength is usually about 0.5 T, though there is variation above and below this value.) Once inside the strong magnetic field, protons within the patient's body water all change their spin to align with that of the magnet's field. (Normally the spins are all in different random directions.) Radiofrequency coils are then used to apply energy to various parts of the body. As the radiofrequency field is switched on and off, the protons in the vicinity of the coil emit energy which can be used to image the organ.

To prevent interference from outside radiowaves, the whole system is shielded within a Faraday cage.

All furniture and partitions near to the scanner must be constructed of non-magnetic materials, and screws, where required, are of aluminium or brass.

Hazards

Powerful magnetic fields of these strengths are not believed to be particularly hazardous physiologically, but the experiences with ionizing radiation have made us extremely cautious and there is little or no information about overdose victims or long-term effects. Mechanical hazards are of enormous concern, however (see below).

Emergency access to patients

During MRI, access to patients in an emergency for resuscitation is difficult whilst they are in the tunnel. All personnel must be fully conversant with emergency procedures to withdraw a patient quickly from the tunnel.

Claustrophobia

For many patients the greatest problem in undergoing MRI is claustrophobia. Recent designs where the patient is not totally enclosed helps reduce the problems experienced by many. Technological aids such as spectacles which allow the patient to see outside the tunnel, as well as music and space-age adventure tapes all help. The experience of some patients within the magnet tunnel is of lying in a coffin – a terrifying experience.

Thorough reassurance and good preparation are vital for all patients, and can make the difference between a successful and an abortive scan. Sedation or even general anaesthesia may be necessary for highly anxious individuals.

Physiological hazards

Thresholds have not yet been accurately defined. Strong static fields may reduce aortic blood flow, increase blood pressure, cause cardiac arrhythmia and impair mental function. Large-gradient magnetic fields may stimulate peripheral nerves and muscles, including cardiac muscle. Heating is a major consequence of exposure to the radio-frequency (RF) pulses used in MRI, and can cause elevated body temperature in patients. With patients who have reduced ability to control body temperature, such as babies, children, pyrexial patients and pregnant women, temperature monitoring should be used. Respiration monitors should be used when imaging babies. All monitoring devices need to be of graphite or other non-ferrous material.

Mechanical, magnetic and thermal hazards

The main dangers associated with MRI installations are mechanical, for example ferrous metal objects flying into the centre of the magnet (scissors and stethoscopes), and partly due to the heating effects on metal objects. Ferrous oxygen bottles should never be taken near to the magnet.

Aneurysm clips, foreign bodies, and implants can become dislodged or heat up, burning local tissues. Pacemakers can be upset and fail under the effects of the field. Digital watches, credit cards, tube tickets and other magnetic materials can be affected by the field.

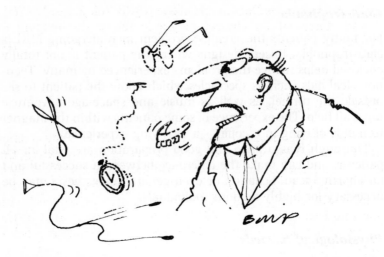

Patients with suspected foreign bodies such as metallic fragments must not be allowed into the scanner; the fragment could become dislodged and cause serious local damage, e.g. the eyeball can be ruptured if a foreign body within it is displaced.

Some types of shotgun pellets are non-magnetic and thus may be scanned safely, but a replica must be carefully checked for movement in a phantom before risking injury to a patient who has one embedded within the body or skull.

Cables used within the magnetic field may cause burns if loops form.

Cosmetics and tattoos

Some types of cosmetics containing metallic powder may be hazardous in the field, either due to heating and burning of the skin or piercing the eyelid under the mechanical effects of the field. It is thus wise to ask female patients to attend for the scan without make-up.

Some tattoos contain ferrous metal pigments; such patients should be advised to notify the operator if a burning sensation is experienced.

Great care must be taken to protect patients from these somewhat unexpected hazards. Staff may also be subject to a no-cosmetics rule if required to work close to the field.

See for reference: Documents of the NRPB Vol. 2, no. 1, 1991, Board statement on clinical magnetic resonance imaging in diagnostic procedures, and User's Handbook, International General Electric, 1990.

Electromagnetic fields

Electromagnetic fields such as those near overhead power lines (and some home appliances) are suspected of slightly raising the risk of leukaemias, breast, brain and prostatic cancers. This is not yet fully accepted by scientists. The mechanisms of such cancer induction (if any) is totally different to that seen with ionizing radiation, where DNA breakages are believed to be the cause of neoplastic changes. With weak electromagnetic fields, this is not the case.

One theory suggests that the normal movements of calcium ions within cells is disrupted by the magnetic field, damaging membranes. Another theory suggests that the earth's magnetic field, which is beneficial to cells, may suffer interference under certain geometric orientations of a weak electromagnetic field.

This could explain why the measured biological effects are difficult to reproduce, only appearing if the geometry is right. Other theories suggest that electromagnetic fields could interfere with organ function whilst leaving individual cells unaffected.

One researcher (Wilson, 1991) has found that weak electromagnetic fields interfere with production of melatonin, a hormone which enhances the immune system, inhibits tumour growth hormones, such as oestrogen and prolactin, and can directly retard tumour cells. Melatonin suppression could well be a risk factor for breast, brain and prostate cancers. The fields are thought to raise the risk in susceptible individuals, though not necessarily cause cancers in the population generally. Men who work in transient magnetic fields may show a slightly increased risk of breast cancer.

Conclusion

This chapter has been rather frightening, yet to put these tiny risks into context we must look again at Chapter 3, and stub out our cigarettes, use the zebra crossing, say no to alcohol and chocolate, fasten our seatbelts and slow the car down before the risks of these hazards even approach those of our everyday lives. (Brent 1989)

Appendix of useful addresses

Health and safety advice

Health and Safety Executive
Secretariat
Baynards House
Chepstow Place
London W2

See telephone directory for local office.

Note: Always seek advice from your RPS or RPA in the first instance:

Our RPS is ....

....

Our RPA is ....

....

Additionally:

National Radiological Protection Board
Chilton
Didcot
Oxon
OX11 0RQ

Tel: (0235) 831600

(NRPB also supply personal dosemeters and a calibration service)

NRPB publications are obtainable through HMSO, see telephone directory.

Radioactive materials advice

For accidents involving spill or loss of radioactive material

HM Inspectorate of Pollution
Department of the Environment
Room A501, Romney House
43 Marsham Street
London SW1P 3PY

Tel: 071 276 0990 ask for senior Radiochemical Inspector.
Outside office hours, ask for Resident Clerk on 071 276 5999.

(Outside the capital these matters are dealt with by local offices.)

Applications for ARSAC licences and advice on nuclear medicine investigations

ARSAC Secretariat
Department of Health
Division HS1A
Room 515/6
Eileen House
88–94 Newington Causeway
Elephant and Castle
London SE1 6EF

Tel: 081 972 2000 extension 22719

Transport of radioactive materials

The Transport Radiological Adviser
Department of Transport
Radioactive Materials Transport Division
2, Marsham Street
London SW1P 3EB

Tel: 071 276 5050

Publications and meetings on radiation protection and quality control

Institute of Physical Sciences in Medicine (IPSM)
P.O. Box 303
York YO1 2WR

Tel: (0904) 610621

Accidents involving X-ray equipment

In the first instance contact the RPA and your regional X-ray engineer. After consulting them contact:

National Reporting and Investigation Centre (NATRIC)
Department of Health
Medical Devices Directorate
Room 413
14 Russell Square
London WC14 5EP

Tel: 071 636 6811 extension 3030 ansaphone 071 637 1674

If the accidental exposure exceeded the guideline multiplying factors indicated in the chapter on overexposure, the Health and Safety Executive must be informed.

Bibliography and further reading

Books

British Institute of Radiology

Docker M F and Duck F A (eds) (1991) *The Safe Use of Diagnostic Ultrasound*, British Medical Ultrasound Society, London

Fendel H, Schneider K, Kohn M M et al. (1989) Specific principles for optimization of image quality and patient exposure in paediatric diagnostic imaging. in B M Moores, B F Wall, H Eriskat et al. (eds) *Optimization of Image Quality and Patient Exposure in Diagnostic Radiology.* British Institute of Radiology Report 20, 91–101, London

Garrett J A, Gifford D, Harvey M J et al. (eds) (1988) *'British Institute of Radiology Handbook', Assurance of Quality in the Diagnostic X-ray Department*, London

Moores B M, Stieve F E, Eriskat H et al (eds) (1989) *Technical and Physical Parameters for Quality Assurance in Medical Diagnostic Radiology: Tolerances, Limiting Values and Appropriate Measuring Methods.* British Institute of Radiology Report 18, London

Moores B M, Wall B F, Eriskat H et al. (eds) (1989) *Optimization of Image Quality and Patient Exposure in Diagnostic Radiology.* British Institute of Radiology Report 20, London

Paris A (1989) Reduction of dose using asymmetric intensifying screens in the diagnostic imaging department. in B M Moores, B F Wall, H Eriskat et al. (eds) *Optimization of Image Quality and Patient Exposure in Diagnostic Radiology.* British Institute of Radiology Report 20, 167–9, London

Smith S, Spencer N M, Faulkener K et al. (1989) Effect of automatic exposure control on patient dose. in B M Moores, B F Wall, H Eriskat et al. (eds) *Optimization of Image Quality and Patient Exposure in Diagnostic Radiology.* British Institute of Radiology Report 20, 198–200, London

Taylor C, Cowen A R, and Wilson I J (1989) Patient absorbed doses in digital subtraction angiography. in B M Moores, B F Wall, H Eriskat et al. (eds) *Optimization of Image Quality and Patient Exposure in Diagnostic Radiology*. British Institute of Radiology Report 20, 200–2, London

Thilander A, Bjurstam N, Eklund S et al. (1989) Optimization of image quality and patient absorbed dose in mammography. in B M Moores, B F Wall, H Eriskat et al. (eds) *Optimization of Image Quality and Patient Exposure in Diagnostic Radiology*. British Institute of Radiology Report 20, 110–12

Zankl M, Petoussi N, Veit R et al. (1989) Organ doses for a child in diagnostic radiology: comparison of a realistic and a MIRD-type Phantom. in B M Moores, B F Wall, H Eriskat et al. (eds) *Optimization of Image Quality and Patient Exposure in Diagnostic Radiology*. British Institute of Radiology Report 20, 196–8, London

National Radiologial Protection Board (available through HMSO)

Medical Radiation 1991 leaflet in NRPB 'At a glance' series

National Radiological Protection Board (1991) Board statement on clinical magnetic resonance imaging in diagnostic procedures. *Documents of the National Radiological Protection Board*, vol 2 no 1

National Radiological Protection Board (1988) *Health Effects Models Developed from the 1988 UNSCEAR Report*, NRPB - R226

National Radiological Protection Board (1987) *Living with Radiation*, 3rd edn

National Radiological Protection Board (1992) Protection of the patient in X-ray computed tomography and further statement on radon affected areas. *Documents of the National Radiological Protection Board*, vol 3, no 4

National Radiological Protection Board (1990) *Radon Questions and Answers*, leaflet for the general public

National Radiological Protection Board and the Royal College of Radiologists (1990) Patient dose reduction in diagnostic radiology. *Documents of the National Radiological Protection Board*, vol 1, no 3

Shrimpton P C, Wall B F, Jones D G et al. (1986) *A National Survey of Doses to patients Undergoing a Selection of Routine X-ray Examinations in English Hospitals*, NRPB - R200

Institute of Physical Sciences in Medicine

Brennen S E and Putney R G (eds) (1984) *Dose Reduction in Diagnostic Radiology*. Conference Report 42 (Proceedings of a meeting, London, 1983)

Faulkner K, Cranley K, Starritt H C et al. (eds) (1990) *Physics in Diagnostic Radiology*. Report 61 (Proceedings of a workshop, Newcastle upon Tyne, 1988)

Faulkner K and Wall B F (eds) (1988) *Are X-rays Safe Enough? Patient Doses and Risks in Diagnostic Radiology*. Report 55 (Proceedings of a workshop, Manchester, 1986)

Goldstone K E (ed.) (1991) *Radiation Protection in Nuclear Medicine and Pathology*. Report 63

HPA Topic Report 32, Part III (1981) *Measurement of the Performance Characteristics of Diagnostic X-ray Systems used in Medicine. Part III. Computed Tomography X-ray Scanners*. Hospital Physicists Association, York

Law J (ed.) (1981) *Practical Radiation Protection Dosimetry*. Conference Report 34 (proceedings of a meeting, London, 1980)

Moseley H and Haywood J K (eds) (1987) *Medical Laser Safety*. Report 48

National Protocol for Patient Dose Measurements in Diagnostic Radiology. 1992, NRPB, IPSM and College of Radiographers

Shrimpton P C, Wall B F, Hillier M C et al. (1990) UK CT practice: aspects of QA and patient dose. IPSM meeting: *QA Update: CT and NMR*, Salford

Wall B F, Harrison R M and Spiers F W (1988) *Patient Dosimetry Techniques in Diagnostic Radiology*. Report 53

The College of Radiographers

Connett R (1987) *A Survey into Radiation Dose Received by Staff Working in Angiography Suites*. HDCR, Module F Thesis, London

Osborn S B (ed.) (1986) *Radiation Protection Supervisor's Handbook*, London

Unsworth M (1988) *Methods of Dose Reduction during Barium Enema Examinations*. HDCR, Module F Thesis, London

Legislation and statutory documents

Administration of Radioactive Substances Advisory Committee (ARSAC) (1988) *Notes for Guidance on the Administration of Radioactive Substances to Persons for Purposes of Diagnosis, Treatment or Research*

Department of Health, *Health Circular H.C.(89)18* (1989), London

Department of Health, London:

The Ionizing Radiation (Protection of persons Undergoing Medical Examination or Treatment) Regulations 1988. HMSO (also known as POPUMET)

The Ionizing Radiation Regulations 1985. HMSO

The Ionizing Radiation Regulations 1985. Approved Code of Practice. HMSO

The Ionizing Radiation Regulations 1985. Guidance Notes. HMSO

Health, safety and welfare at work regulations, 1974, HMSO, London

Miscellaneous

Court ruling against Cornwall and Isles of Scilly Health Authority giving compensation for failure to warn a breast-feeding mother about radio iodine therapy. *Daily Star*, 9 April 1991

Department of the Environment (1991), *The Householder's Guide to Radon.* 2nd edn, HMSO, London

Draper G (ed.) (1991) *Socio-economic Leukaemia.* Office of Population Censuses and Surveys Series, SMPS no. 53, Studies on Medical and Population Subjects

Forster E (1985) *Equipment for Diagnostic Radiography*, p. 113, MTP

Gyll C (1987) *Radiation Protection in Paediatric Radiography*, ISRRT Newsletter, 23, no. 2

Gyll C A (1985) *A Handbook of Paediatric Radiography.* 2nd edn, Blackwell Scientific Publications, Oxford

Gyll C, Blake N S, Thornton A (1986) *Paediatric Diagnostic Imaging*, Butterworth-Heinemann, Oxford

Hawkes N, Lean G, Leigh D et al. (1986) *The Worst Accident in the World. Chernobyl: The End of the Nuclear Dream*, Heinemann, London

Hawkins S and Turner R (1989) 'The Radiologist: A Protected Species?', unpublished conference poster

Health and Safety Executive (1992) *Guidance Note PM77: Fitness of Equipment Used for Medical Exposure to Ionising Radiations*, HMSO

Henderson M, Dawson J, Morgan D et al. (1990) *The BMA Guide to Living With Risk*. 2nd edn, The British Medical Association. Penguin. London

International General Electric (1990) *IGE Signa 1.5 Tesla, User's Handbook*

Myers M (ed.) (1988) *Core of Knowledge Course Handbook*. Hammersmith Hospital, Department of Physics and Diagnostic Radiology, unpublished

Saunders P (1988) *Radiation and You*. Commission of the European Communities, Brussels

Steele H R and Temperton D H (1992) *Patient Doses Received during Digital Subtraction Angiography*. BIR Poster handout. Regional physics and protection service, Queen Elizabeth Medical Centre, Birmingham

Sumner D, Wheldon T, and Watson W (1991) *Radiation Risks: An Evaluation*. 3rd edn, Tarragon Press, Glasgow

Swallow R A, Naylor E, Roebuck E and Whitley A S (eds) (1986) *Clark's Positioning in Radiography*. 11th edn, Butterworth-Heinemann, Oxford

The Royal College of Radiologists (1989) *Making the Best Use of a Department of Radiology. Guidelines for Doctors*. Royal College of Radiologists, London

Wilks R (1981) *Principles of Radiological Physics*. Churchill Livingstone, Edinburgh

Wilson B (1991) Untitled article in the *New York Times Medical Sciences*, 2 April

Overseas publications

Committee on The Biological Effects of Ionizing Radiations (BEIR) (1989) *The Effects on Populations of Exposure to Low Levels of Ionizing Radiation: 1989*, National Academy Press, Washington DC

Comparative Carcinogenicity of Ionizing Radiation and Chemicals. National Council for Radiation Protection and Measurements, NCRP 96 (1988), Bethesda, MD

Gorson R O, Brent R L, Moseley R D et al. (1977) *Medical Radiation Exposure of Pregnant and Potentially Pregnant Women.* National Council for Radiation Protection and Measurements, NCRP 54, Bethesda, MD

Ontario Ministry of Health (1987) *The Healing Arts Radiation Protection Guidelines. HARP Act.* Ontario, Canada

Poznanski A K, Dunbar S, Grossman H et al. (1981) *Radiation Exposure of Paediatric Patients.* National Council for Radiation Protection and Measurements, NCRP 68, Bethesda, MD

United Nations Scientific Committee on the Effects of Atomic Radiation (UNSCEAR) *Sources and Effects of Ionizing Radiation: 1977, 1982, 1986 and 1988,* Reports to the General Assembly, New York

Williamson B D P, LeHeron J C, Poletti J L et al. (1985) *A Glossary of Physics, Radiation Protection and Dosimetry in Diagnostic Organ Imaging.* National Radiation Laboratory, Department of Health, New Zealand

Journal articles

Baldock, C, Arnold, M T and Simmons, S P (1990) Low dose chest radiography – a review of the Philips Pulmo Diagnost 100. *Radiography Today,* 57, no. 644

Balver S, Sones F M and Brancato R (1978) Radiation exposure to the operator performing cardiac angiography with U-arm systems. *Circulation,* 58, 925–32

Banergee B and Das R K (1991) Sonographic detection of foreign bodies in the extremities. *British Journal of Radiology,* 64, no. 758, 107–12

Boothroyd A E and Russell J G B (1987) The lead apron: room for improvement? *BJR,* 60, 203–4

Brateman L, Gordon-Bowers W, Reed-Dunnick N and Doppman J L (1979) Transport protective barrier for fluoroscopy during angiography *American Journal of Radiology,* 133, 945–5

Brent R L (1989) The effect of embryonic and fetal exposure to X-ray, microwaves and ultrasound: counselling the pregnant and non-pregnant patient about these risks. *Seminars in Oncology,* 16, no. 5, 347–68

Consumers Association (1991) Our X-ray survey. *Which?* Jan., 40–1

Ginsberg J S, Hirsh J, Rainbow A et al. (1989). Risks to the fetus of radiologic procedures used in the diagnosis of maternal venous thromboembolic disease. *Thrombosis and Haemostasis*, 61, no. 2, 189–96

Hall E J (1992) The gene as a theme in the paradigm of cancer. *BJR*, 65, congress 68

Huda and Sandison (1986) The use of the effective dose equivalent H_E as a risk parameter in computed tomography. Short communications. *BJR*, 1236, 6

Hufton P et al. (1987) Low attenuation material for table tops, cassettes and grids: a review. *Radiography*, Jan./Feb. 1987

Lotz H, Ekelund L, Hietala S O et al. (1987). Low dose pelvimetry with biplane digital radiography. *Acta Radiologica*, 28, Fasc 5, 577–80

Moores B M (1990) X-ray protection. *Rad Magazine*, Oct.

National Radiological Protection Board (1990) ICRP 1990 - ICRP 60. A summary of the draft recommendations of ICRP, 1990. *Radiological Protection Bulletin*, Apr., no. 111

National Radiological Protection Board (1991) ICRP recommendations – what happens next? *Rad. Prot. Bull.*, May, no. 122

National Radiological Protection Board (1988) Leader article, NRPB guidance on risk estimates and dose limits. *Rad. Prot. Bull.*, Jan.

National Radiological Protection Board (1989) Leader article, Radiation risks and the 1988 USCEAR report. *Rad. Prot. Bull.*, Jan.

Nishizawa K, Maruyama T, Takayama M et al. (1991) Determinations of organ doses and effective dose equivalents from computed tomographic examinations. *BJR*, 64, 20–8

Panzer W and Zankl M (1989) A method for estimating embryo doses resulting from computed tomographic examinations. Technical Note. *BJR*, 62

Rogers and Mathews (1986) X-ray field collimation in diagnostic radiology. *Rad.*, July/Aug.

Shrimpton P and Wall B F (1983) Comparison of methods for estimating the energy imparted to patients during diagnostic radiological examinations. Letter to the editor. *Physics in Medicine and Biology*, June

Shrimpton P C, Jones D G and Wall B F (1988) The influence of tube filtration and potential on patient dose during X-ray examinations. Scientific Note. *Phy. Med. Biol.*, 33, no. 10, 1205–12

Smith M L (1986) Guidelines for breastfeeding following maternal radiopharmaceutical administration. 'Nuclear Medicine Communications', 6, 399–401, *Rad Mag.*, Oct.

Suramo I, Torniainen P, Jouppila P et al. (1984) A low dose C.T. Pelvimetry. *BJR*, 57, 35–7

Index